The Back Doctor Secrets

Written by

David Tennison

The age of the cause

Let's us pause, for the cause,

For that is where the problem's stored.

The symptom is misleading,

It leaves us crying and pleading,

For the sake of our well-being,

Give us the antidote,

Which is seeing and believing.

~~~

With special thanks:

Julie Hamilton

Paula Henley-Cragg

Patrick Hogg

Michael Ralls

Alisdair Stevenson

Melissa Toleman

Family and friends

Foreword

Do we understand our mental health?

I am a registered mental health nurse with nearly 39 years' experience, working within the NHS, mainly with child and adolescent mental health services (CAMHS). I also worked for several years working with adults that had severe and enduring mental health problems. I am a non-medical prescriber, which means I am trained to assess mental health and I can prescribe medication as required.

I'm also trained in dialectical behavioural therapy (DBT), cognitive behavioural therapy (CBT), family therapy, with a master's qualification in primary mental health. With this blend of skills I've had the opportunity to help many people as individuals, families and group sessions.

When I'm assessing an individual's mental health concerns, I often look at their core beliefs and identify the thoughts that are worrying them, as in my experience, this is more than likely the cause. Most patients are unaware of how their thoughts and feelings result in physical responses, which can lead to pain or discomfort. A shift in perspective can create a positive emotional response which can help patients improve their mental health.

How we perceive a situation will dictate what we feel. An example is let's imagine, we are invited to a party. For some people the thought of going to a party will excite them, therefore they will experience a feeling of joy, for others this thought, will cause anxiousness and they will experience feelings of self-consciousness. They could all be going to the same party but the way they perceive the party, will cause a physical effect on their bodies, depending on how they feel. When we understand that emotional distress is due to how we perceive the world, coupled with an understanding of the how our bodies function, we understand ourselves better.

I often find that people are unaware their health is being affected, as a result of their emotional distress, such as:

- sleep problems
- poor dietary habits
- lack of exercise
- Problems with social interactions

They are also often unrealistic about medication, believing that if they are prescribed medication, they will be instantly cured, which is from a culture that people presume, they will be placed immediately on prescribed medication in the first instance. It's understandable that if a person is self-harming or suicidal, they and those around them will be concerned and they will want the quickest route to helping them. However in my experience, medication can cause further distress, due to their side effects, therefore it isn't always the 'instant fix' that people imagine.

Medication is helpful when mental health difficulty is severe and enduring. I will always supplement prescribed medication with recommendations to routine (structure of the day) and therapy sessions. If patients follow this advice I find that their doses required, are less than those that do not follow them, increasing the likelihood of those that do not, to become reliant on medication, both psychologically and physically. With young people I've worked with in the past, they told me that anti-depressants take a while to work, once they do, they feel disconnected from themselves, describing it like living life through a movie.

With young people I prefer to teach them the cycle of thoughts and emotions and how they both affect each other and cause physical responses in the body. In my experience mental distress is often confused with a major mental illness. I would explain to patients that our response to a situation is normal if we feel sad because we lose a loved one, then it's absolutely appropriate to feel this way. Grieving is a natural process that we must go through in this situation. Only when the time we feel sad is prolonged or when it's negatively affecting our lives, should this cause concern.

I designed the Caveman story that David has adapted and is using as an illustration in this book. It is a tool I use to help young people and adults understand that their emotional triggers, affect them physically. With this understanding they can become self-aware, effectively acting as their own therapist. Where possible I use these techniques before considering prescribed medication.

As a nurse I've been required to be vaccinated with the flu and hepatitis vaccine annually. More often than not the flu vaccine has made me feel unwell, although I am still required to take the vaccine. I stopped taking the hepatitis vaccine 8 years ago because I wasn't making enough antibodies.

When I studied for my masters, my research was about identifying low mood and self-harm in young people. We set up a program to identify young people that would benefit from early invention for emotional difficulties. To run alongside this, we set up a support for parenting sessions, to help them understand their children's emotions and at times, challenging behaviour. This was a long-term project of prevention through education.

The project was ironically scraped at short notice to implement a vaccination program to young people in schools (HPV vaccine).

Paula's ideal healthcare system

Based on my experience, if I could wave a magic wand, these are changes I would like to see in healthcare. The system would be built around preventing emotion distress and mental health problems before they begin.

These recommendations would be offered to everyone:

- Teach people how their body functions (what thought and emotion do to the body)
- Parent-child relationship education
- Mindset coaching (beliefs can heal)
- Relaxation and mindfulness
- Education of healthy eating/cooking
- Education of sleep and routine
- Education on hygiene
- Education on the importance of exercise

Regards
Paula Henley-Cragg

PREFACE

Writing a book in 8 month is by no means a task to be taken lightly, as I can attest to. I didn't do it all on my own as I enlisted help from friends along the way. I was surprised how interested they were in this project from beginning to end. I spent a lot of time with them discussing, arguing, and agreeing on the nuances of the topics we will cover in this book. I'm grateful for their time and patience in helping me to formulate my ideas into a coherent message that is in the intended spirit of the book.

In the beginning the plan wasn't to write a book but instead make individual essays. Once they were all there it felt natural to combine them together. Which gave them a deeper meaning and so the book became more than the sum of its parts. The further into the project I got the more I felt the book became and is a piece of art to me. I've spent an estimated 460-600 hours refining and reflecting on this art project.

I want to say from the start I am not perfect. I've had periods in my life when I've not followed lifestyle advice and the last thing I would want is for this book to come across as being preachy or that I am holier than thou. I have habits that could be considered vices, for instance a lot of caffeine went into the creation of this book. I've been known to enjoy a drink on occasion and I intend to celebrate with a cigar on completion of this project. I hope this directness about myself shows, that the message of this book is not about perfection, but is about being authentic with yourself and others.

This book is about living a consistent principled life with honesty at the centre, which in the long-term will empower you.

A trip down memory lane

My Mum is a life-long devout Christian. I've always respected her discipline and tolerance for others, I noticed through observation, the strength believing in a religion gives someone. My siblings and I attended church every Sunday during my childhood. I was even an altar boy for a period, which gave me a sense of purpose. I loved getting dressed up into the uniform, but my favourite part, like most boys was the opportunity to ring the bell to signify the significance of the ceremony, when the priest re-enacts the last supper.

I enjoyed most subjects, but my favourite lessons were science and maths. I liked how these subjects were exact. An answer was found by following a formula that resulted in a definitive answer, it seemed the opposite to religion, which required a faith of intangible concepts. Numbers made more sense to me. The syllabuses were honest and in my opinion, morally correct. My science teachers were always open to ideas and they taught us not only the facts but also the conflicting hypotheses, from which we were encouraged to draw our own conclusions.

Since then I've realized that the most definitive answer to a formula isn't always followed by healthcare and governments, mainly due, in my view, to the politicization of science. In the real world science is used as a unifying philosophy (a belief system), shoe horned to solve all society's abstract problems. In school science was creative but in the real world it's frowned upon to be creative within the political-scientific box.

My route to discovering holistic principles has been unusual to say the least. I left school and joined the Royal Marines; I served in Afghanistan, Iraq and Northern Ireland. In the military I gained a lot of life experience, which wasn't without consequences, I had been mentally affected, I knew friends that suffered serious injuries and sadly some had lost their lives. I did 6 years and 11 months service before I left for 'Civvies Street'.

I was unaware of the divide between medical science and alternative therapies at this point. In fact I didn't vaccination. I vaguely remember fellow students talking about this beforehand, fearful of them and the handlers reassuring them everything would be ok. At this point in my life I had no reason to question vaccines. I trusted this was in my best interests.

When I was student Chiropractor I attended a seminar and one of the talks was on vaccines. I remember having a mental reflex, immediately viewing this with scepticism. I thought they were all mad and I was wondering what I was getting into. However the points they made were clear and plausible.

I didn't think too much of this until by coincidence, I was on another seminar in 2010 and it was announced that a research paper on vaccines and autism had been retracted and the doctor involved was being attacked and discredited. It made national news and was on radio, TV and in newspapers. My fellow colleagues were very cynical about this result, they were adamant this was corruption on large scale. I myself wanted to believe in the honour that this couldn't and wouldn't happen, especially in the UK, although it did seem strange that they waited 10 years before retracting this peer reviewed paper.

As mentioned in the past I've had vaccines myself, in the Marines, I had a vaccine for anthrax because there was a threat of chemical warfare when we travelled to Iraq. As I learnt more about holistic health it wasn't that I thought vaccines were ineffective or dangerous, it was in fact, that I felt there were better choices available to protect myself from potential infections, such as through diet and lifestyle.

I also want to make clear I am not against vaccines. There is clear evidence vaccines can suppress certain infections that cannot be eradicated such as measles. Along with conferring immunity they make some people feel safer therefore; they also give the intended recipient the benefits of the placebo effect which is explained in chapter 1.

I am merely opening a taboo subject that is difficult for people to discuss because the subject is complex and emotive. I want to make something that is complex, simpler for those that would like to learn more about health. I realize the topics in this book will mean I am putting a target on my back. I fully expect to be attacked and discredited from those that stand to profit from this status quo to remain, as they do with anyone that opposes them. I believe all philosophies are valid but if I had to pick one over all the rest then I'd choose utilitarianism, which means any actions is justified as long as it's in the interest of the greater good. I believe I'm acting in the greater good by writing this book and if that means it's going against the grain then so be it.

Hopefully you can see from what I've written here, I didn't just wake up one day and feel this way. My views came to be through study, trial and error and maintaining an open mind. I am blessed that I've had a diverse life, giving me the opportunity to live life through different perspectives. I was very sceptical of holistic philosophy in the beginning because of the conventional wisdoms that dominate our culture, but once you've seen the truth it's difficult to turn back.

Life led me to working in a field that it's impossible not to see and recognize the power of healing that comes from within us.

Regards,
David Tennison

Author's Notes

In this book I am offering health suggestions however this is not medical advice. If in any doubt regarding suggestions in this book, please seek advice from a primary care practitioner for individual needs.

This is an opinion based book on the learning's of my life and experiences. It is going beyond conventional science as it is known today, which is materially determined and therefore limited. It is perhaps the science that was once known but has faded almost into insignificance to be dominated by profit making institutions. It is a science based on the collective, long time acquired knowledge of all of us – common sense.

Our senses are our superpower yet we are progressively relinquishing their power and succumbing to traditional science and its limiting paradigm as an inferior replacement. The truth is we all possess the power we need to save ourselves, within us. We use our senses to make judgements and decisions, this will protect us from harm. This book is about reconnecting us with that common sense and enabling us to make better decisions related to our physical and mental wellbeing.

This book is a protest to the inconsistent, arbitrary rules forced upon us in 2020, which feel more like reversed common sense. In my opinion this is a result of 60 years of dominance of pharmaceutical companies, over health sciences and medicine.

This strangle hold by pharmaceutical companies on not only healthcare but society is causing the general public to lack:

- An understanding of how the body works
- An understanding of how disease manifests
- Denying us personal responsibility over our health
- And knowledge of our health

This book is mostly common sense, that deep down, we all know. Any information in this book can be found from internet searches, or reading newspapers reports over the past six months and books that I've cited in the text. I am merely attempting to connect the dots for all to see.

I want this book to empower normal people, so I've purposefully left out a bibliography of references and where possible, I've avoided using technical language.

David Tennison's Holistic Principles:

- The power that makes the body heals the body
- Our bodies are interconnected parts that combine to be more than the sum of their parts
- Symptoms are signals from the body to let us know there is problem
- Ignore or mask the symptom and the problem will only get worse or take longer to heal
- Resolve the cause, resolves the symptom
- Our beliefs, thoughts and emotions dictate our physical health (health comes from within)
- Diet and lifestyle are more powerful than medication for chronic diseases
- Prevention is better than the cure (proactive instead of reactive)
- Belief in higher power is good for our health and guides our lives to a higher purpose

The Back Doctor's

Three Pillars of lifestyle modifications;

- Exercise
- Diet
- Mindset

Table of Contents:

Introduction

One Friday morning at the beginning of January 2019, I admitted myself to hospital feeling unwell with a fever that was getting worse. I had been volunteering on a Vipassana mediation course when I started feeling ill. I thought this was due to something I'd eaten because I had vomited.

I left the course prematurely on the Thursday lunchtime and drove home feeling that some rest and downtime would allow this to pass. During the night, however, my condition worsened. I found it impossible to sleep, I was unable to regulate my temperature or effectively replace my fluids.

In the early hours, I decided that if I felt the same way in the morning, I would seek help. By 6 am my condition had worsened still and my temperature was rising. I made my way to the local hospital, where I vomited immediately upon arrival. The medical staff carried out tests and eventually found I had an inflamed appendix, which made think of uncle that told me a story once that when he was child he burst appendix when he was walking to school during world war II.

I was told I was a 'medical emergency' and needed to be transferred to another hospital for an operation to remove my appendix. I was given intravenous fluid and two different types of antibiotics. This combination

1

together with knowing the cause put me at ease and I then felt in safe hands.

When I arrived at the second hospital by ambulance, the doctors were keen to take me straight into surgery. This made me feel uneasy. The diagnosis and prognosis seemed to have been conducted in such a rush and I was having doubts that this was the best course of action for me. I briefly discussed my concerns with the doctor in charge of my case and he told me this was the only solution. I felt I was not in control of my health. By a twist of fate the surgery was not scheduled that night. I was transferred to a bed in A+E instead.

There was no doubt about how sick I was. By the time I had reached the second hospital I could feel my temperature rising again and felt completely exhausted. I was given more fluid and antibiotics which brought my temperature down but seemed to drain me even more.

Later that day, I was moved to the cardiac ward as there were no available beds in the surgery wing. The other patients in my ward were mostly elderly and suffering with serious conditions. I stayed there for two nights, the first of which was a blur of fluids, antibiotics, and frequent monitoring by the nursing staff.

On Saturday morning, the surgeon who was operating that day came to see me. He carried out the rebound test (pressing on my appendix to check for pain and inflammation) and told me he would fit me in for surgery as soon as possible. I still had reservations about this but at this stage I had no energy to contest.

I was physically and mentally exhausted. I didn't feel like eating, although I wasn't allowed anyway because I was due for surgery, I could only manage small sips of water, I didn't feel like reading or watching anything. Instead, I just lay there resting, until the next time a nurse came to check on me.

On Sunday there was an improvement. I still felt ill but I was more alert and my reservations about the operation returned. I wanted to know all about my options. The surgeon did his rounds and I discussed this with him. He dismissed my concerns by repeating a rebound test – which was very painful – to further prove his point.

I had been given two types of intravenous antibiotics over the previous 48 hours. There was no doubt I was feeling better but it wasn't clear to me if I was getting better naturally or if I needed to continue to take high doses of antibiotics. I discussed this with the nurse who was polite but very insistent that these were needed for me to get better.

There were occasions when it seemed as if I was being met with hostility for questioning the treatment and prognosis. I decided I wanted to take a lower dose of antibiotics so that I could assess the part they were playing in my improvement. My intuition – which I trust – was apprehensive about this treatment. This caused quite a commotion on the ward. The nurse came back

3

from talking on the phone to the doctor and attempted to pressurize me into taking the full dose. I refused.

It was clear from my scans that I had an inflamed, but not a burst, appendix. I was getting better, therefore no longer a medical emergency. It seemed strange to me that my prognosis was not constantly being reassessed.

That afternoon I did some research of my own and found the evidence to be conflicting as to whether an operation is needed for an inflamed appendix. A burst appendix like my uncle had requires an emergency operation, but not always for an inflamed appendix, also there is a risk of infection from the surgery and a six-week recovery time.

I also learned that the common belief that the appendix is useless and serves no function is false. The newest research shows that this tiny organ is used to store bacteria for the gut, much like a little store cupboard or a natural pharmacy to aid digestion.

That evening I did some serious thinking and decided to place myself in surrender to my body. If I was no better in the morning then I would have the operation but if I continued to improve, I would decline. I laid there meditating, moving awareness around my body and focusing on healing.

It took a lot of energy, focus and determination. I was programming my mind to heal my body. Within three hours, my temperature had reduced significantly, I still felt terrible but I'd just had appendicitis, not eaten for 4 days, and been pumped full of drugs. This small victory was all the incentive I needed to believe that what I was doing was the best for me.

New nurses appeared on shift that seemed to feel that they were the new enforcers to make me take the full dose of antibiotics. They told me terrible stories about how if I didn't take them I could die. One went further by telling me her daughter had died because she never took her medication. I did not question this to avoid offending her. I simply highlighted that my temperature had reduced and that I was feeling much better.

The next step was to try and eat something to see if I could manage to hold it down. I ate some bread with jam and waited patiently. At no point did I feel nauseous which encouraged my convictions that my condition would improve without needing to have an operation. However, in the middle of the night, I was moved to a ward that prepares patients for surgery.

The next morning, a consultant appeared with his understudy and I explained my situation, the research I had done, and how I was apprehensive about an operation. The understudy was adamant I needed surgery and that I could die if I didn't. The consultant, however, dressed him down by saying the final choice was mine and that I shouldn't be coerced into an operation. He told me the newest research in the British medical journal, showed there were marginal differences in effectiveness of surgery, when compared to conservative intervention for an inflamed appendix.

This was a huge relief. For the first time since I had arrived in hospital a person in authority wasn't persuading me that I needed an operation or to take more medication. He listened to my reservations and instead of continuing with a planned operation, he respected my opinion and allowed me to make my own health choice.

On Monday I was discharged from hospital with oral antibiotics. I went home, rested up for a few days and I did some research on herbal remedies. I took these instead of conventional medicine and within a week I felt much better. The problem with my appendix did not return and my body had effectively healed itself and avoided an operation and its risks. This sequence of events dramatically changed the way I viewed the healthcare system.

Now I'm not saying that everyone should stop taking their antibiotics. There is no doubt that antibiotics saves lives in critical and emergency care. My instincts told me the cause was the change in diet I adopted on the meditation course, therefore after I was stable; I decided to make dietary changes instead of taking antibiotics.

It's well known antibiotics can cause digestive issues as they not only destroy unwanted bacteria but also destroy good bacteria (probiotics) that aid digestion. On this occasion I made a decision to switch to natural remedies and it was the correct decision for me. I could only make those calls because I had an understanding of how the body works holistically and because I am in-tune with my body.

All the medical staff who handled my case were kind-hearted and professional, but it made me realize how disempowered doctors and nurses are when making decisions away from the protocols of synthetic medication because of the reactionary nature of healthcare. They do an extraordinary job by providing treatment and care for those who become sick year on year and need medical intervention. However, in my experience they have a disease centric view of health and lack a holistic understanding of the mind, body, and spirit connection.

I found that they were only interested in the shortest way to alleviating my symptoms which was to douse me in strong medication, regardless of their side effects and remove my appendix without considerations to the cost of my long term health. I understand appendicitis can be a potentially life-threatening condition. I can also understand why they would want to remove the appendix in certain situations especially in the eventuality that the appendix was to burst.

I understand emergency care is paramount in saving lives but I felt they lacked individuality to my case. Once it was clear my life wasn't in danger then other factors could have been considered earlier such as my age, fitness levels, diet and emotional health. These were important factors that could have made my prognosis specific to me. At no point did anyone ask me for these metrics other than my age.

I was not asked if any personal triggers could have been a factor in my illness, neither was I asked about my diet to understand if I was nutrient deficient. There was no investigation into the cause of my inflamed appendix. The long-term risks of taking antibiotics were never mentioned nor any risks involved with the removal of my appendix.

This book aims to help others understand that the current treatment plans and prognosis employed by the health system are not the only way to treat disease. I say this with no vested interest in pharmaceutical companies or authorities that stand to benefit from this unquestioning belief in modern medicine.

There's no doubt that synthetic medication is incredibly effective at saving lives in emergency care. My question is their efficacy in chronic conditions. There is a risk-reward every time we take a pill. In a lifesaving situation the reward outweighs the risk. However when we take medication for chronic conditions, although they seemingly make us better by reducing symptoms, over time if we continue to take them, they will make our internal environment toxic.

That is why people are not advised to take anti-inflammatories and painkillers long term. Synthetic medication produces a fast response in the body, that can reduce symptoms, but this comes with a consequence, ultimately affecting our long term health.

Is it all about reducing symptoms rapidly? Should it not be about what enables the best long- term results for a patient, with the minimum amount of side effects? Synthetic medication is the go-to for a plethora of infections, diseases, and conditions but is there an alternative?

The body is more like a plant than a machine. Human beings are blessed with consciousness that is our thoughts feelings and emotions. We are living organisms that depend on our environment, social connections and emotions. We are a connected part of the universe, not something that has been made or designed. Our mindset and beliefs are more powerful than we realize and are just as important to the healing process as the medication prescribed.

May 2020

We are now in our tenth week of an enforced lockdown in the UK against the novel coronavirus, Covid 19. The liberties and freedoms of nations have been taken away, in the guise of protection us against a 'killer virus'. Our chiropractic clinic closed along with retail shops, restaurants, pubs, gyms and schools. Life was put on hold and the world was gripped by fear through governments and the media. We are told that the only way to restore our freedoms is through a vaccine, which we are being assured will be safe and effective, even before any trails begin. How would they know this? Vaccines on average take a four year process to develop not four months. There is something very disconcerting about this situation.

The government has committed £300 million to develop a vaccine while most other trials for new treatments have stopped indefinitely to focus on finding a vaccine. Excess deaths have gone through the roof (currently 15,000/number people that are dead as a result of lockdown) because people needing emergency care were not able to access the NHS.

During this period of isolation, I decided to write a book about my views and experiences of holistic medicine, pharmaceutical medicine and intuitive approaches to health. You might be surprised by the alternative truths that I will present in this book. As a collective, we lack knowledge and empowerment regarding our health and this means that we give our power away to others.

October 2020

As this book is about to go to print, we are about to begin a second lockdown, justified again by modelling of the worst case scenario. We've had plenty of time to plan for this over the last six months to build extra capacity within the NHS and set up a shielding service so that another lockdown could be avoided. Throughout the summer the prime minster was adamant that another lockdown would not go ahead because of the conviction in his policies, comparing lockdown to a nuclear deterrent; let's hope we never go to war!

A rise in normal healthy people being infected is only a problem if the virus is spread to more vulnerable groups. Based on this the government is wrong to place further restrictions on civil liberties, unprecedented in peacetime and would be best to focus on more specific actions to the information available. The government can be forgiven for acting with impulse in the initial outbreak as this was a novel virus; however 10 months later, when so much more is known (especially that the average age of mortality of Covid 19 is 80-88 years of age/higher than average life expectancy in UK!), to still be working from a reactionary nature cannot be forgiven.

To ban activities with obvious health benefits like the gym and all outdoor sport is illogical and does more harm than good. Clusters of council gyms are on the brink of closing, never to reopen because of this decision, along with many other businesses. People in the autumn of their lives being told they must not see their grandchildren, regardless of their individual circumstances. This will and is affecting millions of people's wellbeing as well as a feeling of hopeless about the future.

Lockdown 2.0 is a knee jerk reaction by the government with no measure of knowing if it's successful or not (i.e. there is no measure of how many lives can be saved and therefore deemed a success). Our culture is being possibly being changed forever, by the whims of a few cabinet ministers that are making the rules up as they go along. How much of this unacknowledged and unmeasured tinkering with our culture will affect us is unknown.

A patient of mine is a pub landlord and he has been forced to shut with the prospect of never opening again, even though hospitality contributed only 5.18% of Covid 19 cases from 9th July to the 18th September according to Public Health England figures. In the week commencing the 18th September when pubs (night trade) accounted for 3% to transmission of Covid 19 cases, a curfew at 10pm was brought into place. However educational settings in the same week amounted to 44% of total cases. I'm not saying close schools, colleges and universities, but to close pubs and restaurants and keep education settings open, 'it just don't make a lotta sense' (quizzical Texan accent).

He told me a story that hit the point home for me, that over the summer he had some Italians guests staying at the pub; they were so excited, taking pictures, why? Because pubs likes of ours and the environment they create are unique to our culture. Pubs, restaurants and hotels, are already on small margins, how long can they survive in a world that is not conducive to their business models? There is no doubt we will miss them if these parts of our culture are lost. We will be judged by future generations likely to be worse off, as the people ruled by a government that followed a sunk cost fallacy to suppress a flu virus (the common cold) at the expense of killing parts of our economy and culture.

Even one year ago to consider that the world would be changed to this extent would be unthinkable, but now this is the only future anyone can see.

Be your own authority

Knowledge is power. The more knowledge we gain the better health choices we can make for ourselves and our loved ones. Through this book, I want to give you basic knowledge and understanding of how health works, so that if you are faced with a health dilemma, you can think critically through various options and not be limited to just one.

This book has six chapters that can be broken into bite-size chunks on individual topics or can be read continuously from beginning to end. The first part of the book focuses on how internal and external forces affect our health. Once we have the basic information, we can bolt on further pieces that otherwise would have less meaning. I will show how a lack of knowledge about health leaves us at the mercy of people and institutions that may not have our best interests at heart.

1. Chapter 1 explains what health is and why it's important to understand, in the same way we

regard our finances. Also the different modalities of thinking towards health systems.

2. Chapter 2 talks about vaccines and how modern medicine sometimes gets it wrong. I will compare the unwritten history to the version of history we have been taught and show the disparity.
3. Chapter 3 will show the unnecessary panic and hysteria caused, when these flawed theories have been adopted.

The second part of the book will be about how you can help yourself. There is a doctor inside all of us, the innate wisdom that we all have as human beings. It is important to listen to others but it is also important to listen to you. Your body is always talking to you and once you are able to listen, taking control of your health becomes much easier.

I will suggest alternative medicines which are contrary to popular belief;

1. Chapter 4 will educate you about movement and why it is so important to your general health and well-being.
2. Chapter 5 explains how your choice of diet can either cause or heal disease.
3. Chapter 6 will be about meditation and how you can heal yourself through the power of your mind.

By reading my book, expect to be taken out of your comfort zone, especially if you are only used to viewing

PART ONE

A Caveman Story

Many thousands of years ago there were 'Cavemen'.

They communicated in different way to how we communicate today.

Today we use clever words to describe our thoughts and feelings.

Instead back then they would rely mainly on their body language and tone.

Trusting their instincts was a way of life and is what in many cases kept them alive.

The Cavemen lived in what could be considered a more simple life to that of today. There were no phones or digital technology to keep them occupied, which was probably just as well, as they lived in a world that was more dangerous to that of ours! There were animals that wanted to eat the caveman such as the sabre-toothed tiger. When the Cavemen came into contact with the tiger their instincts reacted quickly to either run away or confront the tiger.

Caveman was an omnivore which meant he was able to eat not only nuts, seeds, fruits and vegetables but also meat, therefore the tiger was not just a threat to this hunter/gather, he was also food. In the age of the Caveman there were no shops to buy food, so this would also be an opportunity to feed their family. The Caveman was excellent at recycling as when they defeated a Sabre-tooth tiger they would use the bones for tools and the fur for clothing.

This is called the flight, flight or freeze response or the survival response and this is still relevant to us today.

This is when the innate will to live inside all of us causes a chemical reaction to release adrenaline into the blood stream to muster a mass of energy that otherwise would not be available to us, to survive and protect ourselves and our loved ones. Although today, in our modern world we do not need to face Sabre-tooth tigers anymore because our world is safer than it once was. We also are able communicate in more sophisticated language, which can diffuse situations without the need for conflict. However this prehistoric chemical response still happens, when we perceive a threat, are worried or stressed, real or imagined. Here are a few examples of how we may describe this:

- ❖ Anxiety
- ❖ Panic
- ❖ Impulsive acts
- ❖ Nausea
- ❖ Sore throat
- ❖ Red mist
- ❖ Palpitations
- ❖ Stomach upset
- ❖ Headache
- ❖ Tears
- ❖ Fuzzy or dizzy feeling

- ❖ Shaking
- ❖ Fist clenching

The Caveman would only ever use the survival response for short duration and then their body would switch back to rest, digest and restore, which is the opposite of flight or fight. This is when the body recovers from a surge in adrenalin into the blood stream. However what if the Caveman couldn't switch off the survival response because they were in constant fear of a perceived threat such as a Sabre-tooth tiger. When we are in a survival situation, it's normally not only stressful, but also highly emotionally charged, therefore being stuck in fight or flight is exhausting and will likely affect how our body functions, which eventually will cause signs and symptoms in our health.

Chapter 1: What is Health?

"The biggest mistake physicians make is they try to cure the body without curing the mind first"

Plato

Part 1: The Sickness Model vs. The Holistic Model

Health means different things to different people. To your GP, health is more than likely the absence of pain and disease, which means that when we are free from pain and disease, we are considered healthy. This is a common belief within the medical profession, who generally believe that when we are not displaying any symptoms, there is no reason for you to see them.

They work firmly on an evidence-based model, meaning that nothing is real unless it can be measured, quantified, and proven. However, what if this model was built on a false assumption and is now limiting medical progress and understanding of health and illness? What if there was an intervention that was self –evident but its research was not recognised because other methods were taking precedent?

You generally visit your GP when you experience pain or symptoms, although when does disease actually start? Does it begin when you receive a diagnosis? Modern medicine would like us to believe that disease appears as a result of our genetics, family history and / or environment. However, the cause of disease usually develops over time, due to many reasons that in most cases are preventable.

When you see your GP, the appointment time is short. Whenever I've ever visited a GP they've focused on my symptoms and resorted to a generic pool of pharmaceutical medicine to prescribe as a solution. If I was in pain they prescribed pain killers, if I had an infection they prescribed antibiotics. They were focused on eradicating the symptoms with little consideration to the cause (outside of a few tick-box questions around lifestyle/vices).

Medical practitioners are generally mechanistic in their approach throughout their careers which stems from their training. This means they deduce answers by focusing on finding and eradicating the symptoms of the disease as the solution without addressing the underlying cause. This is a reductionist philosophy involving solely rational, mechanistic and isolated viewpoints, removing other possible factors such as a person's beliefs.

For this reason medical practitioners will only consider biological responses and discount the influence of thoughts, feelings and emotions on our health and wellbeing. As such, treating us like a machine that can be serviced into good health. We are, however, more plant than machine and in treating our ailments we need to take a more holistic and preventative approach to self-care as we might in taking care of a garden.

Imagine instead of watering your plants in your garden regularly, you waited until they started to show signs they were dying before tending to them. It makes sense to be proactive in a garden especially if you want your plants to live long and be healthy. Wouldn't this also make sense that healthcare was proactive, instead of waiting for us to become sick? Tradition medication could then be used as a final resort should disease develop despite holistic efforts, instead being used as a first port of call.

In my own personal case, the doctor's recommendation was to have my appendix removed, which would have undoubtedly relieved the symptoms – problem solved. Only I would have been left with fewer organs than I walked in with and more importantly, the underlying source of the issue was not considered, investigated, or addressed. Whilst my body was trying to tell me something, I was being viewed and assessed only by mechanistic measurements and solutions.

Chasing symptoms

It seems logical to me that stress could be a cause of high blood pressure and I have met many patients prescribed medication at the very first sign of a raise in their blood pressure. They take prescribed medication, their blood pressure is reduced and their symptoms disappear, however, if stress was the cause in the first place, have they successfully solved the problem, or are they just masking the symptoms?

Symptoms are the body's signs telling us we are out of balance. If we mask the symptoms with medication the cause of the problem will not be solved, which in turn makes the body fall further out of balance. This invariably leads to further health complications and more medication. This is the problem with the 'treatment of symptoms' - it does not seek to identify the underlying cause of the symptoms. The underlying cause could be a number of things, including an emotional issue or a dietary imbalance.

Let us take another patient who is suffering with high cholesterol and anxiety. More than likely the patient would be put on separate medication to control each one of these symptoms. I have known patients to be prescribed statins for high cholesterol and antidepressants for anxiety. After successful completion of the prescribed course of medication it may appear that the problem is solved. But if it hasn't addressed the cause, the patient will continue to live the same lifestyle and the imbalance will remain, or even get worse. The medication will have only masked the symptoms, leaving the lifestyle or emotional imbalance that caused the issue to continue to wreak havoc with the patient's overall health. Therefore the conventional solution in this scenario means that these medications are taken for an indefinite period.

When statins were first introduced, they were only given to those with an existing cardiovascular condition, however they are now recommended to anyone over the age 50, regardless of whether or not they are suffering from high cholesterol. They are used as a preventative measure against developing high cholesterol and resultant heart and cardiovascular diseases, as lifelong medication. However there are side effects to taking statins, so immediately there is a trade-off between the 'possibility' of reducing the risk of cardiovascular disease and also putting a person at risk from taking the medication.

My view is that pharmaceutical medication should be the last resort after all natural remedies and solutions have been explored. Modern medicine has strayed too far away from our nature as a result of its quest to solve all our health problems with an outside in perspective and artificial means. This is supported and sponsored by the investment powerhouses that drive our healthcare advancements.

There are three 'wonder drugs' in our society that are too often overlooked by the medical profession as a result of its reactionary nature. And whilst there is a general awareness of these 'wonder drugs', we as a society have yet to fully embrace their power and ability to contribute proactively towards a long and healthy life. What are these drugs? Exercise, diet, and mindset.

If doctors recommended lifestyle changes before, during and after their patients were sick they would be more likely to follow the advice. Most people trust and respect their doctors, often without even questioning their advice. The doctor is in a position of knowledge and power to help their patients take long term, preventative strategies through which the patient can assume responsibility for their own health. When someone knows how and why they are doing a task, not just the mechanics of it, they are more likely to achieve the best results and stay committed. This means doctors working with patients to create long term health strategies from early on in life.

Altering your lifestyle can have a big and very positive impact on your health, and there are no side effects. It begs the question: is taking conventional medication better than implementing lifestyle changes? Perhaps we should simply ask ourselves: does health come from a pill or does health come from within us?

When the term health is used in a holistic context, it refers to a living being that has inter-connected parts which all affect each other and cannot exist independently of the whole, or indeed be understood without reference to the whole. That's to say our body and our health is in fact more than the sum of its parts, and each part cannot be looked at in isolation of the rest, as a means of diagnosis. Holistic health is viewing the person, as a whole, by taking into account their biology, mental health and social factors, rather than just the symptoms of the disease. When a patient is treated holistically, these background triggers are assessed as possible causes of the symptoms – treating the cause and in time, clearing the symptoms. This is the difference between proactive and reactive care.

After my experience of the current health care model, I realized the difficulty in making judgments on our health is because most studies are based on factor changes within the body that negate a holistic approach. The science shows that the drug made a change and is therefore effective, whereas holistic changes happen on an interconnected level, individually and collectively contributing to an impact that is larger than the sum of its parts, but difficult to measure using modern preferred methods.

Currently the health system treats the body like a machine, breaking the parts down into isolation to explain the whole. We are living organisms that are created from small beginnings, we have the ability to grow and reproduce. How many machines can do that? To build our health system around the machine principle is to take a very limited view on health.

Under these assumptions we are constantly moving away from nature's natural laws and adding flawed mechanistic theories. In doing so we misunderstand the natural world we live in; that we are just one of its many parts. These ideas do not stop at pharmaceutical medicine they extend throughout our science and consumer culture.

This idea that if we add something to us we will be more or better is seductive. Advertisers know this and they use these ideas to hook us. Artificial sweeteners and low-fat products are a couple of examples where it's implied that if we consume these products we will be healthier. A belief system is created through skilled mass marketing. However, they are gimmicks purely designed to encourage consumption.

This brings us to the Placebo Effect which is our 'belief response' measured as a key factor in drug trials. We already have the understanding that our belief can be so strong that it can positively impact our health. This is why new drugs are only approved if they can beat Randomised Controlled Trials (RCTs) in a double-blind study. This is when the participants are split into two groups and one will take the medication and the other a placebo. The participant and the organizers are blinded to which group is which (if they did know their own beliefs would certainly influence the results). That's to say, our current medical regulation already accounts for the power of the Placebo Effect!

The placebo effect is regarded by science as a measure against a drug however, after its use for this purpose only, is considered irrelevant and disregarded. Yet the placebo effect seems much more important than we appear to appreciate as it clearly demonstrates that a patient's beliefs and hopes play an important part in the healing process. It shows our thoughts, feelings and beliefs can determine our recovery from illness. It's clearly an integral part of the healing process, so why isn't it considered when treating patients? When truly understood, cultivated, trained and honed, the beliefs in our mind can be far more powerful than anything that can heal us externally.

Your beliefs determine your health. A hypothetical example of this, imagine two people have identical life threatening cancers, with 'weeks to live', the doctor tells them the prognosis, the first patient says "that's it, it's over", but the second says "I'm going to empower myself to overcome this", which one is likely to live longer? It's seems clear to me that the mindset of the second person is more likely to live longer than the first person who feels apathy and resignation.

What would happen if either of these patients started to address the life situation that was the potential cause of the illness?

The exclusion of metrics that cannot be tested in a RCT such as our behaviour and motivations are limiting our healthcare system. This tunnel vision approach is shaping how medicine is being taught to future doctors, and the policy makers that fund research, which are strongly influenced by the powerful pharmaceutical companies whose primary concern is to make large profits for their shareholders.

An integrative model that widened the scope for therapies to be included, by using comparative effectiveness research would be able to factor in lifestyle metrics, which are impossible to test under double blind RCT conditions. In this way the power of the mind could be used in conjunction with conventional synthetic medication to heal people faster and more effectively.

Much as our beliefs can set us free from the limited views of modern medicine. The current health system is based on a limiting belief system, which censors the information that is made available and imprisons us within its boundaries (a reactionary disease centric model of healthcare). It could be said that modern medicine's current belief structures appear to better resemble religious dogma than truth seeking inclusive science.

Here are some thoughts on what modern medicine's 10 commandments might look like:

1. Do not question vaccines or their effectiveness they are our saviour that has wiped out diseases of the past (they are the only answer to controlling and preventing disease. Anyone that dares to question them is to be attacked and condemned)
2. We will wait for people to get sick before acting (we will avoid listening to attempts to make a proactive healthcare system)
3. The body is a machine and consciousness is an illusion (we will only recognise consciousness as the placebo effect)

4. The medical model is the only model (all others that cannot be incorporated into this narrow view that the body is a machine, are to be deemed inferior and useless when compared to the might of the medical model such as chiropractic/homeopathy/acupuncture)
5. We will pick and choose the evidence that suits us (We will move the scientific goalposts to accept what suits us)
6. The placebo is an unwanted consequence in drug trials (we will refute that the placebo is an integral part of healing)
7. We shall escalate to synthetic medication before any natural interventions
8. We will put people on lifelong medication regardless of the side effects (they are the only solution)
9. We will be the patsy's (yes man) to the pharmaceutical priest's 1 trillion dollar industry
10. The body doesn't heal itself, our treatment plans and drugs do that
11. Disease is an enemy to us (we must use confrontational/war language when describing it instead of understanding that the disease is part of us)

I got carried away with this list and produced 11 instead of 10. Not to be taken too seriously of course!

At present we go to see external doctors so that they can tell us how we are feeling, when what we really need from them, is helping us understand what we are feeling. Doctors of the future will teach us how to understand our own health so that we can take more responsibility of our lives. In this future doctors would be there to coach, subtly teaching their patients.

The doctors of the past were Sharman or priests, chosen because they would have been the smartest integrated person in their community. They would have had a mix of principled philosophy, science, human psychology and deep understanding of nature. Intuition would have been their most powerful tool.

Doctors of the future will be hybrid practitioner's that will help individuals understand their own situation and formulate a strategy to overcome their issues before any medication was prescribed. The focus will be on tracing the problem back to the cause.

What if everyone was offered a consultation session with a medical professional at periodic stages of their life to check in with them, in a similar way newborns goes for check-ups? We could continue this for every developmental stage and then every 1-3 years from adulthood to old age, regardless if they are displaying symptoms or not.

What if we viewed health the way we view other subjects, such as English, maths and science? The concepts of health taught to students and adults, on how to make better choices, could prevent many diseases.

Healthcare could be just the start of a wider change in society. A world that is centred emotionally by the majority of its participants will likely to cultivate beneficial habits and behaviours for the greater good. All that's lacking is awareness this is possible. If we believe, we are one step closer.

That is the power of possibility, when we understand the difference between the symptom and the cause, we can acknowledge our mistakes in real time, to reflect and learn from the cause.

Part II: What makes us Healthy?

"Perception is awareness shaped by beliefs, beliefs control perception. Rewrite beliefs and you rewrite perception. Rewrite perception and rewrite genes and behaviour".

Bruce Lipton

The branch of science called epigenetics has revolutionized how we view health over the last 30 years. In the beginning epigenetics was met with extreme scepticism but is now an accepted science of the biology of cells.

You may be surprised to know that our genes are not pre-determined as we have been led to believe. Pre-epigenetic science said that our genes controlled our destiny. In this theory we were victims to our genes because if a parent or relative has or had heart disease, then we were warned we may develop the same condition.

Instead, is it a self-perpetuating manifestation, more likely to come true because we believe it to be so? This common cultural belief is engrained into society that we are less powerful than our genes can be comforting for some, but scary for others, who feel they are unable do anything about their fate. However is it really true, does this predisposition exist or is this just a belief?

The DNA within our genes has a characteristic unique to us, they determines our makeup such as the colour of our eyes. If you have ever watched a child grow up, you will know they have traits and ways of being that they were born with, which no one ever taught them. There is no doubt that nature plays a huge part in who we are but how much does our environment, ways of conditioning and the choices we make, shape us as individuals?

Inside all of us are 70-100 trillion organized cellular universes, mainly consisting of water and minerals. At the centre of each cell is a nucleus, which is considered to be the cell's reproductive factory. This is where our blueprint (DNA) is kept. Think of the nucleus as a huge library, which contains your genetic code.

Anything perceived in the environment through our senses such as smell, taste, warmth and cold gives a mirrored biological signal to every cell. Without external stimuli the cell remains unchanged. Whatever is being sensed by the human, is directly affecting the cell.

The outside membrane of the cell has protein antennas, which sense the environment and determine the function of the cell. If for example a hormone is sensed externally, proteins bind to each another to open a gateway, allowing the hormone to enter, much like a key turning in a lock.

Epigenetics has proven that the membrane of the cell is the equivalent of the brain and not the previously thought nucleus, at the centre. The nucleus reacts to the cell membrane that delivers instructions to the cell for gene production and not the other way round. Genes are not self-activated, which means a particular gene does not decide if it is switched on or not. Therefore how can they determine our reality or our health? The answer is they cannot, but other factors such as environmental triggers can and do influence the expression of our genes.

DNA produces proteins that are selected from information received from the external environment of a cell, meaning the cell is constantly adapting to its environment. The assumption that the cell produces predetermined genes randomly or according to our heritage is no longer a unified theory.

The cell is ultimately determined by our external environment, internal belief systems and our emotional health.

Can you see now that your perception of reality governs the cell? There is no DNA or gene involved when deciding the behaviour of the cell. Only an external stimulus can cause an internal response in the cell or a change in gene production. Therefore, your beliefs will positively or negatively affect your genes.

Your environment, internal perception and diet (what we feed the cells) are what control your genes. By understanding that the fate of your genes is not pre-determined and is largely a consequence of the choices we make, we can start to control our health.

Understanding the body in this way has always made me question marketing campaigns by the NHS or Cancer charities such as "We will beat cancer together" or more recently "NHS, against arthritis". It is clearly important to want to help and develop better interventions for sufferers but is making the disease that is a part of them (rewritten genes) separate from them and something they need beat or kill the best way to help them get better?

This separation of the person from their illness denies them the acceptance of their behaviour as a potential cause of the disease. Would it not be better to understand the cause in the first place, rather than viewing their aliment as an enemy? A person can then start to take responsibly by making the changes needed to overcome the disease or aliment.

These factors which make them susceptible to developing disease are often overlooked in these campaigns. I believe it would be more helpful if they conveyed the message that disease can and is often caused by these factors that go unacknowledged in modern medicine.

When you look out into the world what do you see? Do you see a world where you are master of your destiny or a world where you are a victim of circumstance? The view a person holds will be reflected by their cells behaviour and genetic production, thus making those views a biological reality. For further reading I highly recommend the Biology of Beliefs by Bruce Lipton or You Are the Placebo by Joe Dispenza.

The brain is more malleable than we thought. Through neuro plasticity the brain can change and adapt just in the same way our cells adapt to thrive or survive in their environment. If a person went to the gym regularly and lifted weight they would build muscle. When we challenge ourselves mentally the brain makes connections that are analogous of building muscles by building connections in the brain. This enables us to be able to learn or grasp concepts more easily, solve puzzles or release our creativity. This in turn generates a more positive mindset that will establish itself as our habitual way of thinking.

The fact is, the body has the power to heal itself. Stop and think about that for a moment. When you cut yourself or break a bone what heals you? Your body does. We all have the ability to heal ourselves naturally when we are healthy. This is side lined by medical reductionism because of the belief in the effectiveness of pharmaceutical medicines to solving isolated symptoms in the body.

It is in my opinion that your beliefs can literally make you healthy and they can make you sick. Your beliefs can speed up and they can slow the healing process. Your beliefs are more powerful than we are led to believe.

Words have meaning. Words have intention. Words have vibration.

In quantum mechanics the building blocks of life are in a constant flux, vibrating in a wave like formation. The entire universe is in a state of vibration but each and every vibration is unique just in the same way that your fingerprint is unique to you. Everything you touch, every cell, atom, bone or even a stone, they are all vibrating. The reason we cannot see the vibrations is because they are vibrating at an incredible speed of 570 trillion times a second.

Everything in existence has a vibration and when vibrations resonate, they will vibrate simultaneously when in close proximity to each other. For example, if you had two tuning forks of the same frequency, and you hit one fork causing it to vibrate, the second fork will vibrate at the same frequency automatically. Yet if you were to try this with another fork that had a different frequency, there will be no reaction, sound or vibration. Therefore when two things have the same vibration, they resonate.

When we understand that we are vibrating then we can start to understand that our emotions and how we feel also have a vibration. Words make up 7% of our communication; the other 93% is through body language, tone, and the energy we emit.

Most adults have all experienced and recognized someone that is experiencing great sadness – they needn't speak, for us to know this. A person, who is sad, could be crying or hunched in posture, this energy has a vibration that the other person will pick up on. There is the rational explanation that visual cues trigger cascades of signals in the brain leading to the conclusion that this person is sad. However do we only sense through rational means?

We all have the sensory skills to feel the vibrations of others because these skills predate words or analytical language. Our ancestors would have been deeply attuned to these ways of being that have been censored in our culture since the rational enlightenment in the 19th century. These are the sixth sense skills that have not been discovered by science or deemed accepted by the scientific community because of its devout commitment to the reductionist model.

Have you ever heard someone describe a person as if they could: "light up a room"? No words would be spoken but this person would have something about them that others would notice. Could this be because the person was vibrating an authentic joyful emotion that others were drawn to notice? Think about what this person's posture and energy would look like, would they be hunched and smaller in appearance like the person with great sadness or would they upright and appear larger than they are?

A person that has genuine love and gratitude towards themselves and others is more likely to attract others that are vibrating those emotions too. Whereas those that focus on standing on others to feel better about themselves will attract similar energies, therefore we become mirrors of the people we spend time with. When we have a love for life that's not limited to romantic love our frequency is raised to vibrate a love and respect for all beings which in turn attracts people with a similar outlook.

When we vibrate at this frequency we are led by the energy of our hearts and not our heads. We will begin to think of others, ourselves and respect for the planet. In turn this will improve our own lives, providing increased love and gratitude, enjoyment, health and happiness. If we live to please others, feel jealously or self-centeredness, we limit the love and gratitude available to us and in turn more likely to feel sad, resentful and dissatisfied.

Vibrations in the body go through the levels from the sub-atomic, atomic, molecular, cellular, organ to multi-organ that results in a whole being. Just like when tuning forks resonate at the same frequency so too do the levels of our being. It's important we stay in tune with ourselves on all levels so that our body communicates and interacts at its best. When a part of the orchestra falls out of tempo, not only is his part compromised, it will impact those musicians around him. Our bodies work no differently.

When people talk about being on the same wavelength, could this be what they really mean? Emotions and feelings that have a vibration will resonate with another person experiencing the same emotions. As opposed to two people that always disagree or dislike each other. For me the key to resonating with someone is empathy because when we think of the other person's point of view we begin to see the world through their eyes.

Have you ever been with a friend or a partner, someone that you know well and all of a sudden they say something innocuous but the change of tone indicated clearly to you that something had changed in their emotional state. This is an example an when we are in tune with another person, we recognize it immediately.

Words are important but they can also be misleading. For example, if someone was to say thank you, we might assume on face value that they are being genuine but if the intention was not genuine, we would likely sense a tone in their voice and manner. This is why intention and the subsequent vibration they emit is far more important than the words spoken. Once we realize this communication becomes clearer and we can grow as individuals and as a collective consciousness.

To expand on this point I'd like reference the work of Masaru Emoto. He was a Japanese author that worked with scientists studying frozen water crystals. He had a realization that no two snowflakes that ever landed were ever the same and mused could the same be with water. His work was a science experiment that also turned into a piece of modern art. Of his many experiments he found that under a microscope, that frozen water crystals were much more likely to form in water that had a positive vibration compared with water that has a negative vibration. He used many different techniques like playing music to a sample of water but probably the most remarkable was water's sensitivity to words.

In this experiment he wrote positive words (such a love, peace) onto pieces of paper and fixed them facing inward to a cylinder of water. He did the same with negative words (hate, war). Time and again in experiments the positive words formed a beautiful symmetrical shape of crystals and the negative words produced an ill formed baseless shape without crystals. Notably, after water was shown the word "war", no crystals could be found whatsoever. How could water understand or distinguish between the different attachments to the words to form very different outcomes?

My own interpretation is that the words used in this experiment (and their collective meaning) are being mirrored back to us in a 'symbol' in the form of crystal formations; remember we communicated through symbols long before words. Is there something we have lost or forgotten because we rely on words instead of symbols in our modern world view? It an interesting concept and an area I would like scientists to research further so that we can understand more about water consciousness and the collective meaning of words and their intentions.

If this experiment can be replicated then the implications are huge in terms of understanding intention as a force, which in many ways is like the placebo effect we discussed earlier, and why water somehow reflects us and the world around it. If this could be proven science could use water in new types of trials to establish more than we already know about life and this could be a way to understand ourselves and the universe better.

In his book The Hidden Power of Water he asked people to perform their own experiment that can be conducted by anyone at home. They had three glasses of cooked rice and for one month they were instructed to give thanks to the first glass, to the second glass to say 'you fool' and to ignore the third glass. At the end of the month the first glass fermented with a mellow smell, the second glass the rice went black and rotted, and the third glass, rotted faster than the second glass that had derogatory comments. Masaru Emoto drew the conclusion that being ignored was possibly more damaging than being ridiculed.

A study was conducted on plants where one group of plants was shouted out with derogatory comments, and the other group of plants was serenaded with uplifting loving words. In the first group the plants didn't grow as expected, they were misshapen, asymmetrical and smaller than usual. However, in the second group the plants that were treated with respect grew symmetrically, vibrant and larger than the first group. This is an example that the intention of words has an energetic frequency.

The results of this experiment will resonate with any keen gardener out there. Plants grow better when people have a relationship with them instead of viewing them without a consciousness. Many botanists attest to talking to their plants with words of praise to help them grow faster and produce more beautiful flowers.

It's not just plants or humans that are affected by positive energy; places can also have them too. That's why our homes feel the way they do, or places of worship give us that sense of peace we associate with them.

My parents are both in their seventies and a few years ago they went to Lourdes in France which is said to have healing powers. It is said that by drinking the holy water there, miraculous healing can take place. They both said they felt different following the visit and were uplifted for some time afterwards which was a surprise to me as I know them to be sceptical in nature and difficult to convince at the best of times. Again, even if you believe it's only a placebo, my parent's emotional state improved and therefore their health improved.

The Communication Network

Your body has 11 systems that work in harmony together. The master system that links them is the central nervous system (CNS). The CNS consists of long bundles of nerve tissue descending from the brain, down through your spine and extending out to every part of your body. It is what connects 'you' to the rest of your body. Think of the CNS as a dashboard with a number of functions that let us know what is going on. For example, when we feel pain it is a warning signal that there is a problem in that area.

Upon conception, the first part of the embryo to be created is the nervous system which imprints on every part of your body. Think of this as a sensory map of the human body imprinting on your feet, hands, enteric nervous system (digestive system) and many others, connected by the homunculus in the brain. This is how a reflexologist can make a diagnosis about someone's health purely by examining their feet. The feet represent every part of your anatomy, including your organs.

The nervous system is interwoven into the spine from the very beginning because of its importance to survival and function. Your blood vessels travel outside of your spine because they are more elastic than nerves and their function is less complicated than that of nerve function. Anyone who has studied neuroanatomy will tell you how complex and counter intuitive the subject can be.

In most instances, nerves work best by maintaining their length. They are like cables we use for electrical appliances at home and they have very little elasticity. If they are stretched beyond their limits, your body will sacrifice movement by turning on muscles spasms to protect them. Nerves can change length over time and adapt to muscle lengths, which are more elastic and are able to stretch but will resist sudden changes in length.

There are three main functions of the central nervous system: sensation, which makes up 10%, movement making up 30%, and the regulation of organ function which makes up 60%. If I put my hand behind my back, even though I can't see my arm I know where it is in space because I have spatial awareness. I can feel hot, cold, numbness, tingling and many other sensations. If I want to wiggle my finger, an instruction is sent from my brain down through the spinal cord into my arm and all the way to my finger, through a motor nerve which recruits muscles to move my finger.

Organ functions are mainly subconscious and depend on the body's mode (operating system) which we will discuss shortly. If for example your blood sugar levels are too high, subconscious feedback detects this through autonomic nerves signals (neurotransmitters or chemicals governing our brain function) to the pancreas which will release the hormone insulin into the blood stream.

The CNS is sending and receiving these types of messages, some conscious and others autonomic, (subconscious) between your brain and body in every moment of your life. They are literally keeping you alive! For example, take a deep breath in now and you will find that you are aware of your breathing for a moment. However, in time your attention will drift but you won't stop breathing. If you were to hold your breath for an extended period, you would faint before you could harm yourself. The reason for this is because the power of the subconscious is more powerful than our conscious mind.

Growth vs Protection

The modes for the CNS have different effects on the body. They are: 1) fight, flight or freeze and 2) rest, digest and restore. This can also be broken down again into a simpler format: 1) protection and 2) growth. Your body is either in one or the other. It cannot be in both. You are either in protection mode or in growth mode.

Think of the brain as a big computer. The skull and brain are the hardware and the software is our thoughts, feelings and emotions. A computer will only have one operating system running at any one time and this is the same for your body.

An emotional response to perceived external stimuli dictates the mode of the CNS. For example, a person who feels threatened (fearful) is more likely to switch to protection mode. Through subconscious evolutionary processes, your body will be ready to generate masses of energy just to survive based upon instinct in less than a blink of an eye. In protection mode the blood flow is pumped to the limbs, which enables us either to fight or take flight in a survival situation.

However, if you perceive the external stimuli as being comfortable and safe, over a period of time the mode will switch to growth. In this mode, the body will focus on using energy to rest, digest and restore functions such as the removal of toxins and restoring fats, proteins, vitamins and minerals. In growth mode the blood flow is focused to the abdomen and organs.

Being in protection mode is normal for short periods. It is a natural bodily process that was designed to be switched on for short duration to generate energy to help humans and animals evade damage or death. For example, we get butterflies when we look over the edge of a cliff because our body is expressing danger through our organs.

Let us take another example. A lion is lying in reeds stalking a gazelle that's grazing. The lion darts out from a concealed position and is spotted by the gazelle and a chase begins.

To avoid certain death, the gazelle's nervous system makes a split-second subconscious change to protection mode and then a conscious decision is made to take flight. There is nothing more important to the gazelle than evading capture and its nervous system reacts accordingly.

A biological chain reaction begins when neuro-transmitters travel from the brain, down through the CNS to the adrenal glands above the kidneys, which releases adrenaline into the blood stream. This stimulates the heart to beat faster, pumping blood to the limbs enabling the gazelle to sprint faster and for longer than normal.

If survival takes place, rest is then needed to replenish, as being in protection mode uses a tremendous amount of energy. The body needs to restore function by switching back into growth mode. A similar response would happen to us if we did a bungee jump or parachute jump.

Our brains subconscious patterning would release small amounts of adrenaline to a perceived threat to life, even with conscious thoughts overriding that it is safe and in some cases fun. Once the jump was over and we felt safe again, the body would return to growth mode.

However, what happens when we are unable to turn protection mode off?

Humans are so intelligent that they can create their own reality. Your thoughts are so powerful that your mind cannot tell the differences between imagination and real life. Therefore, how we perceive a situation regardless of reality will dictate our biological response.

If we constantly perceive stimuli to be threatening, our brains operating system will switch to protection mode. This is called a sympathetic dominant state (protection mode constantly on). The adrenal system becomes over stimulated and overused – way beyond its short burst duration capabilities, which over time can cause conditions such as fibromyalgia and adrenal fatigue. This is why prolonged periods of stress are so detrimental to our health and a major contributor to disease.

The bottom line is that under stress we shut down our growth mechanisms and this is not limited to dangerous situations. A study compared children living with their parents and children in orphanages. A child that lived with their parents was more likely to develop healthily than a child not receiving parental support.

It appears the more love and support we have as a child the better our development will be. Could this be because we are promoting growth over protection mode. By understanding these modes we can have more control over our health. By recognizing a situation or an emotion that triggers protection mode we can

50

avoid or make a conscious decision whether protection mode is needed.

When we enter protection mode, we are more likely to make reckless decisions than when we are calm and settled in growth mode. I personally delay making a decision that can wait when I am in a stressful situation because I know that when I'm calm I make better decisions.

Stress is part of life. We are constantly under stress from natural forces such as gravity. Stresses in our life do not cause protection mode, our perception of reality does. Protection mode is not something to avoid but it is something that you want to know how to balance and use wisely.

The immune system

There are many reasons why people become sick and in fact having a cold once in a while is good for us, by helping to clear unwanted toxins from our systems. These symptoms are either informative or detoxifying. A temperature for example is result of your immune system working effectively to allow detoxification.

Our immune system keeps us healthy and protected by fighting infections and removing anything harmful from the body. When the immune system is compromised, we become weaker and are less able to protect ourselves. When they are functioning effectively, they are proactive and keep us protected from disease.

Immune responses are linked to the modes of the CNS. When we are in protection mode, survival is prioritized over immune functions, compared to growth mode, when they will take precedent. Protection mode is there to keep you safe from the external threat in the environment. However, the immune system protects you from internal threats. Remember the gazelle? Evading capture was the only thing that mattered in that moment and fighting an infection became insignificant. This means that the body will heal faster when your body is in growth mode compared with protection mode.

Have you ever heard that teachers tend to become sick during the school holidays? They generally carry out a stressful job, which could promote protection mode. When the school holidays begin they relax, the immune responses are switched back on by growth mode and the result is that their body allows them to become sick, as a necessary process of recovery and repair. It is as if their body waits until it is safe to do so.

The immune system is the body's natural house cleaner, mopping up anything unwanted or harmful to the body. It fights new infections with the production of white blood cells (WBC) or if there is memory immunity to an infection, antibodies are released into the system to neutralize and prevent the spread to other people. This can only happen smoothly when the body is in growth mode. If you spend too much time in protection mode, the body is unable to carry out these functions. Put simply, when you have stress hormones in your body, the immune responses are reduced.

The effectiveness of our immune system is strongly related to what we think and feel. When we are happy and healthy our immune system will be more resistant to becoming sick. However, if we are unhappy, run down and fatigued our immune systems are less resilient and more likely to get sick. If you are experiencing negative emotions such as anger, guilt or shame, they all tilt towards pushing your body into protection mode. Positive emotions such as happiness, love and gratitude on the other hand, tilt the body towards growth mode.

Our immune system work best when we receive natural sunlight and have the correct vitamin levels. Sunlight helps produce vitamin D in the body which is vitally important to bone density. A mixture of sunlight and hormones (testosterone in men, oestrogen in women) produce vitamin D. When women go through menopause their oestrogen level drops that's why osteoporosis is associated with women post menopause. When their body produces less oestrogen they lose the ability to convert sunlight into vitamin D. Sunlight also has been proven to be a germicide.

When we have the correct vitamins levels in our bodies they help our immune systems naturally fight infections. For example when a baby is born their immune system is fragile however, breast milk has high levels of vitamin A which has been known to be useful in fighting off childhood infections.

Emotions

The adrenal system functions from fear-based emotions such as feeling scared, angry or frustrated. They are there to dominate other emotions until the threat has ceased. Whereas the autonomic, digestive orientated functions is dominated by love-based emotions such as feeling joy and fulfilment.

When you are in a heightened state of emotions, they are like protection and growth mode, so at an emotional level I call them, 1) Fear and 2) Love. We may seek love when we are fearful however when we are really scared we are focused on surviving, so that we can feel love in the future. Our focus and energy is switched to the adrenal system.

When this happens our digestive functions scale down until safe to resume. This means that fewer nutrients will be extracted from the food we eat, than if we were relaxed. That's why some people get runny stools or the opposite; they become constipated when they get stressed. The digestive system is compromised for protection mode and resources are being redirected elsewhere which has an effect on normal digestion.

Sexual intercourse in general does not use the adrenal system so blood flows to our sex organs instead of to our limbs. In most cases to procreate we need to feel love as opposed to fear. In a state of fear a woman may feel tightness in their vaginas and men's penis' will shrink because of blood flow to your sexual organs will be significantly reduced until the threat has passed.

Some emotions can be sustained for long periods of time and others cannot. If we get scared and need to take flight, our energy resources can only be maintained for a period of time and then the body will need rest. What if the fear never leaves, such as in the case of shell shock? This was a condition first discovered in the First World War when medics realized that suffers were left in a constant state of shock even after the shelling had stopped.

Knowing how to identify, understand and resolve negative emotion is the key to maintaining good health. It's also important to understand that feeling these emotions is normal; there is no need to eradicate them, but instead understand the cause behind them. We are all likely to experience negative emotions throughout a lifetime, but by being gentle with ourselves, we can explore their origin and understand how to resolve them.

When we feel depressed our brain chemistry produces low serotonin and low dopamine however when we are feeling happy our brain's chemistry has normal serotonin and dopamine levels. Every emotion has a chemical balance within the brain and in turn has a mirroring hormonal level in the body.

Taking anti-depressant to improve our emotional state is an option used by modern medicine to resolve depression. Masking difficult emotions has some benefit in the short term but they do not address the cause.

Even when people feel better after taking anti-depressants can be misleading. The person feels better but what if that person was feeling those emotions because of a decision they had made, their emotions had arisen to help them understand their decision. Anti-depressants would have changed how they feel but the likelihood is this person won't have grown mentally or spiritually in the process. Therefore the chance of the problem reoccurring or manifesting itself, in another way will be highly likely.

If you have the courage to face these emotions and understand them, they can be processed and released. At times this might be painful but as they pass you will feel better afterwards. It doesn't mean you will never feel those emotions again but each time they surface you will be able recognize the trigger and manage them yourself. All that's needed is emotional support and an understanding this feeling will pass.

The fact that we feel negative emotions makes us human. When we are healthy and centred we can clear them quickly and as a consequence will feel them less often and with less intensely. When we can balance negative emotions with authentic positive emotions, regardless of our habits we are more likely to be happy and healthy. However, when we feel negative emotions regardless of how well we eat or how much exercise we do, we are more susceptible to becoming sick. Our emotion shapes our world view, which shapes our health.

The information we perceive from the world is neither negative nor positive. We judge it based on our beliefs, principles, experiences and our ability or inability to manage stress. We place a filter over the information to make it mean something to us.

Essentially your emotions and beliefs can vitalize you or they can make you sick and when you are sick they determine how quickly you will get better. If you have an optimistic outlook then your body will focus on your natural healing abilities bestowed upon growth mode, but if you are downbeat with no reason to get better the less likely you will be able to harness your innate self-healing powers. This is why being mindful of our emotional health is as important as brushing our teeth.

Inflammation, the body's cellular scaffolding

Our body uses inflammation when any kind of repair is needed. If you bump your knee and a bruise appears what you're seeing on the skin is internal inflammation. Within the bruise, the body is creating a space for that area to go through a healing process. Imagine builders on a building site (white blood cells/immune response) restoring a site with scaffolding. Once the debris (old dead tissue/blue/brown discoloration on the skin) has been cleared and everything has been replaced (new tissue) the scaffolding can be taken down, as in the bruise disappears.

When we sleep this is the time our bodies' rest and repair. In the first four hours of sleep the body repairs and in the second four hours our minds go through a similar process. Inflammation is an important part of the healing process. However when the body isn't getting enough rest (growth mode) inflammation sites cannot be removed effectively.

Heart disease has been closely linked to poor sleeping and dietary habits, which increases the risk of strokes and other heart conditions. Inflammation in chronic diseases is a reaction to toxins which accumulate in the body from physical and emotional stress and from what we eat. When these illnesses are a result from diet and lifestyle the logical solution is to change them.

Inflammation is part of the healing process so why are we so quick to use over the counter anti-inflammatory medication? When we use these, they remove inflammation, but they also slow the healing process because inflammation is your body's natural scaffolding for repairs. Anti-inflammatory medication does have benefits in the short term but if taken long term can cause digestive issues.

A natural anti-inflammatory is ice applied to the site of the pain or injury. When ice is applied the blood vessels contract to cool the area and then when the ice is removed fresh blood can flow into the area. 'The scaffolding site' can be reduced and more specific to the area where healing is taking place. Avoid using cold gels because they just trick the nervous system that the area is cold which may give pain relief but will not create fresh blood flow that aids healing.

The Breath

The breath is the key to the switch between the two modes. When we are in protection mode our breath becomes short and shallow, breathing mainly from the top portion of the ribs and lungs. Someone hyperventilating is a classic example of a person being in protection mode.

Conversely, breathing in growth mode is relaxed and usually incorporates a long contraction of the diaphragm into the belly. A long intake of breath such as sighing or yawning is breath tilting towards growth mode. Immune and digestive responses turn on, old inflammation can be removed and increases blood flow.

That's why breath work in yoga and meditation are so good for us because they control our state (modes). Through the breath we can clear emotions that sometimes get stuck in our minds. Breathing is the window to our emotions, with each emotion our breath changes. When someone gets scared they might momentarily hold their breath or have a sharp intake of breath, as opposed to when are relaxed they will breathe normally.

By actively changing our breathing cycle with breath work we can change the way we feel. Therefore, if we are feeling anxious, depressed or angry which normally result in shorter, shallower breathing, we can counteract these emotions by actively taking long and deep breaths for a few minutes which is sometimes called belly breathing. With these simple exercises we can change how we feel, just by our breathing.

Posture

"If you would seek health, look first to the spine"

Socrates

When trees are healthy, they will grow upright and symmetrical, and the same applies to us. Therefore, our posture is a good indication of how healthy we are.

The spine isn't one bone it is in fact a collection of bones on top of one another forming three distinct curves. When these curves are in their optimal position, they provide the flexibility and strength needed for their versatile role.

For ideal posture when we look in the mirror your nose, sternum and belly button will be aligned and your shoulders and pelvis will be level. Looking from the side; your ear, shoulder, pelvis, knee and ankle will aligned measured by a plum line or right angle from the floor. Lastly you want all the spinal bones to aligned without leaning or twisting.

Our posture is a direct reflection of how we think and feel. For example, when we are stressed our shoulders raise and become tense, or when we feel depressed our shoulders slump and our head will come forward. Our posture tells us a lot about ourselves and our personality.

When we are in the correct positions we move as nature intends and there is no need for aches and pains. The natural built-in patterns of movement use the correct structure to synchronize balance and coordination to move effortlessly. However when we lose the correct geometric positions the reverse happens, our balance and coordination will become less synchronized with our movements and the structures are more at risk, increasing the likelihood pain and discomfort.

We also adapt to our environment, for example when we sit at a computer for long hours without breaks, generally our heads will come forward from our shoulders and our hip flexors will tighten. Or we sit with one leg under the other for extended periods which causes the pelvis to become unlevel. All of these actions are possible triggers to injury. Over time, the more we adapt away from nature's geometric positions, the more likely injury will occur and/or reoccur.

The cerebellum in the brain is where our balance and coordination is controlled. The cerebellum relies on your spine to move free of restrictions. The longer restrictions are there, the more likely they are to create poor movement patterns that are more prone to injury.

When we have a barrier to optimal balance and coordination such as an injury or restrictions in the spine, the cerebellum will make alternative pathways to cover the loss of the injury, however if the injury or restriction is never fully addressed, this will become a chronic problem therefore, the cerebellum does not fully recover the optimal pathways for balance and coordination. This is a cycle that cannot be corrected until the restriction has been removed.

People can have an issue for many years without pain and then suddenly the body cannot make any further adaptations without damaging a certain area. The body therefore sacrifices movement through muscles spasms and pain to protect the area. The healing time will be dependent on a person age, mindset and other factors.

If someone continues to ignore the symptoms the healing time will be longer compared with someone who recognizes the symptoms. They are not always physical and can also be emotional.

A common solution is to avoid the trigger that causes the problem. Let's take a classic example of a gym exercise that causes pain or injury, so the person avoids this exercise, the symptoms go. Out of the blue they start to feel the same injury on another exercise and then another, and then another until before they realize they are restricted to minimal activity to avoid flaring the problem again. It could be a shoulder, a knee, their lower back, whatever the problem joint is, avoidance was never going to solve the issue.

In the beginning the problem was only there for short periods and then they recovered but as the injury continued to worsen, the time they felt good flipped to experiencing discomfort for a long duration. This reoccurring injury means they start to struggle with basic tasks they took for granted. Not only is the problem getting worse, the situation is also affecting their vitality, self-worth, motivation. Their dietary habits, exercise and mood has all been affected because they made better lifestyle decisions when they were fit and healthy.

It's usually at this point they turn up to my chiropractic clinic or other body worker specialists, seeking advice and help. At what point could they've intervened? Could this problem have been resolved earlier? Think back to the start of this chapter when we discussed modern medicines approach of 'if it isn't broke, don't fix it'. As the general public we've been led to believe the best course of action is to wait for the symptoms to arise before acting and as you've seen from this example, the symptom is usually the tip of the iceberg.

The key is to understand that most injuries are caused by poor movement patterns and incorrect posture. If your head is coming to far forward from your shoulder acting like a counter lever on your lower back, then over time don't be surprised if you get a lower back issue. By focusing on removing poor movement patterns to maintain good balance and coordination before you get injured, will save you a lot of trouble in the long run.

If you correct your posture you will be less susceptible to future injuries. It doesn't mean you will never experience an injury in the future, but it does mean they will happen less often and if they happen the recovery time will be quicker.

The disc

In between each one of the bones is a disc, which is 70% water, acting as a spacer for the nerve roots and shock absorption. When we run we are generating forces 12 times our body weight and this is absorbed mostly through the spine and the discs.

When the spine is aligned optimally there will be an equal amount of space and weight between each one of the discs from the base of your skull to your sacrum (bottom of spine/part of the pelvis) however when we lose the shape of the spine the ability to distribute these forces becomes significantly reduced. For this example let's discuss a car's suspension.

The suspension system in a car has a set of pistons elevated by stretched springs. When the springs are placed under force, the springs compress to cushion the pistons. If the suspension was already compressed when hitting a speed bump there would be less absorption of force, therefore an increased likelihood of damage to the wheel arch.

The suspension analogy helps us understand the disc from a mechanical viewpoint however; the body is a biological organism that has evolved through nature. It is made up of collagen, ligament, and fibrous material. Inside every disc is a nucleus that regulates the discs, mechano-receptors (sensation and pressure antennas). To understand this more let's use a donut as an example.

Imagine a donut was in a vice like force between your hands, the donut could be compressed and returned to the original position however if you were to continue the compressive forces on the donut for an extended period, then the donut would take longer to recover. Now consider placing a donut on a surface and striking down hard on one side of the donut, the jam will be forced from the middle of the donut to the edge of the donut however, if the force is large enough the jam will be forced out of the donut.

This is what can and does happen when someone 'slips a disc'. For example, over time they lose the shape of their spine placing compressive forces onto the disc. This is a serious injury that can be very painful.

You can lose the shape of your spine long before pain is felt. The key here is to act before a structure is at risk, rather than waiting until its debilitating.

Bringing it all together

The body is interrelated by our cells, organs and systems. Each individual part depends on another part to complete their function. When we inhale air from the atmosphere, our lungs diffuse oxygen into our blood stream that is pumped around the entire body by our hearts through the blood pressure in our arteries. The renal and lymphatic systems cleanse the blood of waste products so that once the blood returns to the lungs through our veins, it is ready to be oxygenated again.

When we eat, the digestive system takes the nutrient from food for growth, repair and energy. Waste products are removed and anything that can be of salvage will be stored in the liver and abdomen. The functions of the digestive system, such as hormone release of insulin from the pancreas to remove reduce blood sugar levels will depend very much on what we eat and how we feel.

This is coordinated from the CNS which acts as a communication network for all systems sending messages at several hundred miles an hour. They are like satellites orbiting the earth that could beam back instant messages from across the globe in Australia. Whereas digestive and hormonal responses act like trucks delivering food supplies to a supermarket through the road network of the vascular system.

The nervous system receives a list of what's needed for the shelves and then packages are transported through the blood. This is what's happening when inflammation forms. Your body has decided that repair is needed in that area. All the material needed to heal the area is sent through the blood.

If the communication between the organ and the CNS isn't functioning for whatever reason, the order of what's needed will not match with what's being communicated and therefore the organ may not get what it needs. The body can function in this way, however overtime this will cause some kind of symptom relating to that function or area of the body. When one organ isn't functioning this has an effect on all the other organs because they are interrelated. They all part of the same supply and demand chain.

The white blood cells could be considered as a combination of all three emergency services. When a signal of a problem is received, white blood cells are released from their substations around the body called the lymph nodes. They will cordon off an area and remove anything harmful to the body.

I've used some analogies of our day to day life to tie the body's systems together. They are individual parts of the whole, however like day to day life they have a cause and effect on one another. To understand them we must understand they all depend on each other to maintain what we call health.

Our beliefs, environment and emotions as a consequence of life situations, trigger our cells, organs and systems to react in accordance with them. When we are in protection mode the cells will become defensive, our organs will sacrifice their needs by diverting blood to the limbs. Immune, sexual, digestive functions are all switched off so that the focus of energy is on survival. The opposite happens when we are in growth mode.

These are just a few examples of how the body works and how sometimes the problem can be tracked and traced instead of waiting for symptoms to arrive. There are many other ways that disease manifests and it's an area that needs to gets as much focus at the tail end of when we are sick. The healthier you are the more capacity your body has for healing itself. If a person has an emotional imbalance that they do not address, then eventually they will experience bodily pain or symptoms of dysfunction health.

Chapter 2: Vaccines

Before we begin

This chapter is Pandora's Box, once it's opened you may never view vaccines the same way again. If you are open to an alternative view then please read on however if you know that your views on vaccines are not ready to be challenged then by all means feel free to skip this section of the book.

My goal is to help you become healthier through understanding the effect of our beliefs and emotions in connection to our health. If you have a strong belief in vaccines this section will question this taboo therefore, think carefully before reading. If at present your view is vaccines are absolutely necessary to making you feel safe and protected then counter arguments are likely to cause an emotion imbalance. If this is the case, as I said feel free to skip this chapter.

I would rather you felt safe and centred than challenge your world views when you may not be ready for them. In the last chapter we discussed how our immune system is impacted by our emotions, when fear is perceived the immune response is sacrificed for protection mode. Therefore our immune system is more susceptible to being compromised by how we feel than any other factor.

This chapter will be discussing the history of vaccines, questioning their efficacy. Along with myths such as modern medicines claim that small pox was eradicated by the small pox vaccine and also that other childhood diseases declined because of vaccines. I will also explore the concept that by supporting immunisation programmes, we are in danger of side lining essential lifestyle factors and we are not helping the plight of poorer nations.

"Every time an unvaccinated person enters their office, zealously pro-vaccine doctors arrogantly overlook the truth that the person's risk of dying or being maimed from the accepted medical practice they offer, is far, far higher than any possible death or maiming from the supposedly vaccine-preventable disease."

Dr Barbara Starfield

(Journal of the American Medical Association)

Vaccines- Humanities Saviour Or Pseudoscience?

Finely tuned immune systems vs. vaccines

Human beings have been on this planet for thousands of years. During this time we have lived alongside vast amounts of microbes that have enabled us to develop a fine-tuned, healthy, and effective immune system. However modern medicine actively promotes vaccines, as absolute "necessities" to keep us and our loved ones safe. Unfortunately, in this quest to protect us, there is legitimate taboo question that go unanswered; regarding the effectiveness of vaccines and in some cases dangerous side effects, from harmful substances on an otherwise healthy person.

We are told that vaccines are the miracle of modern medicine. We are advised that they saved millions of lives by eradicating smallpox and suppressing childhood infections like measles As well as protecting the elderly and vulnerable from influenza, claiming to increase our lifespan, and making our lives and those around us safer.

We are told by both the government and medical professions that recommended vaccinations are essential and necessary for our safety. If we refuse them, we are told we are irresponsible or negligent because we are not following the "proven" scientific facts. We are advised that if we do not comply, there is a significant risk of becoming infected and seriously ill, as well as of being a dangerous risk to others by contributing to mass infections of an otherwise controllable disease.

The idea of a vaccine is very seductive. A person is given an injection that allows them to become immune to an infection, which they would likely have contracted through a lifetime of being in contact with other people. This therefore, reduces risks to their health and others due to no longer being contagious and spreading the infection. I have to admit that if it was that simple, I would probably agree. However, when you scratch the surface, it is revealed that reality is often quite different from this original perception.

The vaccine argument is so persuasive that most healthcare systems throughout the western world use immunization program that stretches from the cradle to the grave. When I was born in 1982 only 10 vaccinations were given throughout an individual's lifetime. Today the number is significantly more, with multiple vaccines often being administered at the same time. This includes vaccines with toxic chemicals, and potentially harmful, heavy metal substances (usually needed to stabilize and preserve the vaccine to help improve its shelf life) into a healthy baby, all in the name of protecting them.

The schedule for vaccination is arbitrary and has never been questioned as to its effectiveness. There is very little known about the potential side effects of vaccines when they are administered in close proximity to one another. It has also never been tested for carcinogenesis, mutagenesis, or infertility. We have no idea what the long term consequences of these vaccines are because there has never been a study done to fully investigate this. However, most authorities throughout the world continue to recommend them.

We are programmed to gravitate towards safe options and the vaccination theory feeds off this programming. We are fearful of being unable to prevent ourselves from a long term disability, when in fact it's a paradox because the vaccine could also cause them. We are steered as individuals towards vaccination through the fear of 'what if?' However 'what if' being exposed to the vaccine was more of a risk than the infection itself?

The only measure of efficacy by vaccines is their ability to stimulate the immune system to produce medically induced antibodies. The more antibodies they produce, the more effective the vaccine is considered to be. However, just because vaccines create antibodies linked to fighting infections, the person will never develop whole cell immunity, which is what happens when a person recovers from an actual infection.

The flu vaccination is administered every year to the older generation and those who are most at risk are encouraged to have a vaccination, but despite this 14,000 people still die every year from influenza, including people that have been vaccinated. There have been no controlled clinical studies demonstrating a decrease in influenza after receiving a vaccination; therefore it would appear that the flu vaccine cannot guarantee effective immunity.

Every winter different flu strains spread throughout communities and seriously affect the older population. The medical profession along with the pharmaceutical companies prepares a flu vaccine that contains the most common strain from the previous year. However, bacteria and viruses mutate month to month, year by year, so producing a vaccine to protect people against the correct strain for the flu virus, for that specific year is like finding a needle in a haystack. Is this the most effective way of protecting our older generation?

Originally the flu vaccine was only recommended for people of a certain age with underlying health conditions. Today it is recommended to each age group annually, including infants and school children that have a relatively low risk to any flu strain. How did we digress from protecting the very few at high risk to mass inoculation for everyone?

Vaccines may or may not protect you from flu, however it will expose you to the risk of serious allergic reactions, febrile seizures, or Guillain Barre Syndrome. The majority of flu vaccines use mercury in each dose. Mercury in the blood stream can cause mercury poisoning.

The 6 in 1 vaccine is given at 8, 12, and 16 weeks old to protect against Hib (Haemophilus influenza type b) and other infections. Today, however there are only a handful of Hib cases compared with during the 1980s when 20,000 children every year suffered from this serious infection.

Initially it appears that the vaccine may have been a huge success; however, there is a caveat. The vaccine has removed the risk of type b infections but these have instead been replaced by other strains. One study referenced in Robert Sears, the vaccine book, shows that the number of NON-type b infections amounts to the same number of type b infections that were present before the vaccine was introduced.

Strain replacement is a problem for many vaccines, as they successfully eliminate the targeted germ only for another one to take its place. These new strains can be more dangerous than the original ones because they are more resilient to antibiotics, such as is seen in the pneumococcal and HPV vaccines.

It is unclear whether vaccines can cause autism as the research is both conflicting and controversial. Some believe the potential side effects of vaccines could cause damage to the brain, resulting in autism. Although there is no confirmed link between vaccines and autism, there is however a link between environmental mercury and autism. It is thought that heavy metals passing through the blood-brain barrier could cause brain changes that are linked to disabilities.

Dr. Sherri Tenpenny, a world leader on the subject of vaccines has reported there are 57 peer-reviewed research papers to demonstrate the connection between vaccines and autism. However, this is disputed by the pro-vaccination lobby groups who still maintain there is no association between the two, because of this some parents are confused as to whether vaccines are in-fact safe or not. They ultimately want to protect their children but possible valid research against vaccines is being discredited to encourage vaccinations.

The debate on vaccines is now incredibly polarised and the general belief is that pro-vaccine lobby groups are anchored in scientific proof while anti-vaccine groups are based on unsubstantiated scientific evidence. Governments and pharmaceutical companies are choosing to label any detractors as unscientific or uneducated.

Vaccination court

Parents with limited medical knowledge are left at the mercy of this paradoxical divide because a significant amount of valid scientific research against vaccines is possibly not being recognised. If there is an adverse reaction or unpleasant side effect to a vaccine however, the manufacturers of vaccines hold no responsibility.

The manufacturers of vaccines in the USA cannot be sued or held liable if a person becomes unwell as the result of receiving a vaccine. They have 100% liability protection due to the 1986 national vaccination injury compensation program. So even if a vaccine was to cause death, the manufacturers have no liability. As of 2019, $4.2 billion has been awarded to claimants.

It seems that vaccines receive a lot of protection and are viewed differently to medication. For example if someone were to have an allergic reaction to penicillin, they would wear a bracelet for the rest of their lives, but if someone had an allergic reaction to a vaccine, no precaution is taken to stop that person from having another vaccine. We presume they are for the greater good and the majority of people, including our courts, do not even question them.

Once vaccines are approved, they remain approved, so when one is labelled safe, they are seldomly removed. Most vaccines could be updated, improved, and made safer but this would cost billions of pounds to redevelop them. There is no incentive for pharmaceutical companies to make them safer because they have complete protection for their approved product.

Imagine buying a new car that on purchase was assured by the manufacturer to be safe and effective, but when driving off the forecourt the brakes failed and caused an accident. Under normal circumstances it would be natural to take the issue to the manufacturer, which they would then take responsibility. However what if the manufacturer said it was your fault and denied responsibility and the government not only backed them, they paid out for the company?

History of Vaccines

Vaccines were derived from the process of variolation which begun in China in the Middle Ages. Scabs of smallpox victims were crushed and then blown up the noses of healthy people in the hope that they would become immune to the disease. Acupuncture needles were also used in a similar way to help transmit immunity from an infected person to a non-infected person.

These ideas were further developed by 19th Century physicians, who were able to buy their title and position without any formal training or understanding of current sciences. One of these physicians was Edward Jenner. You may recognise his name from the Jenner Institute which is currently working on discovering an effective Covid 19 vaccine. Jenner's beliefs were never proven and his work is heavily scrutinised by today's scientific standards as being inadequate and unsupported.

His whole smallpox theory was based around just one subject; a boy he deliberately exposed to smallpox via a vaccine in 1796. When the boy did not contract smallpox, Jenner presumed that the vaccine was not only effective but that the boy would have lifelong immunity from the disease which was a false assumption. Jenner was taken very seriously by the government at that time and they would go on over the next 50 years to embark on the first wave of compulsory vaccinations.

Jenner took the variolation principles one step further. He began growing smallpox on cows on a mass scale, funded by the government, collecting the pus from the infection, and injecting into humans, most commonly babies. Many vaccines are still produced by using animals as the host, such as the flu vaccine which is grown in chicken's eggs. However, Jenner's experiment on a mass scale was a failure, instead of becoming immune, many people were infected with smallpox, this not only spread the disease further, but this also meant vaccinated people were dying of smallpox and secondary infections. They were taking a vaccine that was more likely to kill them than confer immunity.

In 1853, the law required compulsory vaccination of every child within three months of birth and by the 1860s, 96% of babies born in London were vaccinated. However, smallpox outbreaks still occurred and in 1871-72 there was a worldwide pandemic that ravished countries throughout the globe. This was the largest seen that century, despite the measures taken by governments to use vaccines in places like Boston, Chicago, England, and Japan.

If parents refused vaccinations, they were prosecuted, but despite the deterrent, many still opposed the law because so many children suffered serious side effects and even death after the procedure. This opposition grew further after the 1871-72 pandemic. There were two prosecutions in 1869 which had increased to over a thousand by 1881. People from all social classes were becoming increasingly sceptical of vaccines due to continued smallpox outbreaks spite of mass vaccination.

Figures taken from London hospitals admissions in 1871 showed that 73% of all smallpox cases had received a vaccine and yet they still went on to develop smallpox. In Germany it was estimated that 1 million people died of smallpox even though they had been vaccinated between 1870 and 1885. People were being vaccinated but they were still becoming sick from the disease. By receiving the vaccine, they not only put themselves at risk of death from the disease but also from the actual vaccine itself.

Compulsory vaccination was not working for three reasons; 1) the vaccine wasn't providing immunity as Jenner's model had previously predicted 2) administering the vaccine could be a lethal injection as there were no sterile instruments and needles would be used multiple times. This resulted in not only deaths due to the vaccine itself but complications due to a secondary infection 3) sanitation was not being considered as the most likely cause of the disease. The compulsory vaccine laws were more likely to start epidemics rather than successfully stop them.

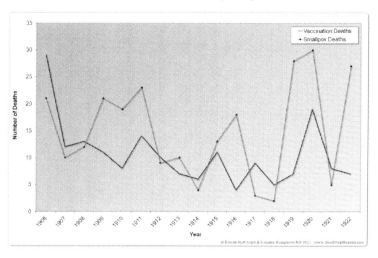

This graph compares smallpox deaths and deaths caused by the smallpox vaccine. This graph like many others can be found in the book 'dissolving Illusion' or can be found on their website www.dissolvingIllusions.com

Sanitation vs Vaccination

The medical profession credits vaccines with successful eradication of small pox, the decline of diseases such as whooping cough and measles, but the statistics clearly state that these infections were on the decline long before vaccines were introduced. So what was the real reason for the fall in infections that ravished our ancestors?

Poor people of the 19th Century would often eat rancid meat along with nutrient-deficient diets that left them highly susceptible to disease. They had jobs that involved hard labour, often working 14-16 hours a day with no minimum wage. Children also worked for long hours from a very young age. This was a notoriously sick and unhealthy era resulting from the conditions people lived in and no vaccine was going to change that.

Vaccines could kill people quicker than any disease due to the lack of sterilisation and hygiene. After arm to arm vaccination was banned, the same needle would be used from person to person, resulting in cross-infection. These were times when medical knowledge and a general understanding of hygiene were limited.

The reason for the decline points towards improvements in sanitary conditions but vaccine companies and the medical profession rarely acknowledged this fact.

Diseases of old declined as our knowledge of sanitation improved. Our ancestors were unwittingly killing themselves by contaminated water supplies as a result of throwing garbage including excrement and dead carcasses into the streets and drains.

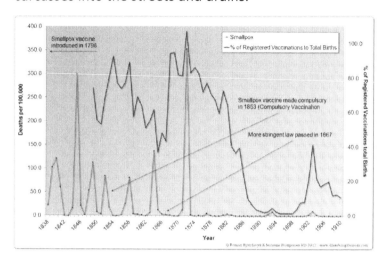

Graph: Top line shows percentage of total births vaccinated. After the outbreak in 1871-72 people's (bottom line) views on what was causing disease had changed. Sewers were built in London (finished 1880's) to separate clean and waste water. Other cities around the world would follow suit.

Coupled with overcrowding, poor ventilation was also a recipe for the rapid spread of infection and disease. The Greek and Roman cities had well-regulated public health systems but this knowledge was somehow lost and only rediscovered in the mid-19th Century with the realisation that contaminated water was causing cholera.

John Snow was credited with discovering the connection between contaminated water and cholera. He realised a well in a London district was the cause of the cholera outbreak. People who drank the water from this well became very sick but the workers of a nearby local beer brewery remained healthy. The workers were given free beer by the brewery and therefore didn't drink the well water and this is how the connection was proven. This was the first time that modern observers considered and took seriously that poor sanitation was the cause of disease.

John Snow however, was ridiculed by his peers at length before his theories were finally taken seriously. The modern microscope had not yet been invented; there was no awareness of microbiology, microbes of bacteria, and viruses. To some, this idea probably sounded like esoteric witchcraft, with the idea of an invisible killer spreading through contaminated water. It took time for others to be convinced but he was not the only person starting to arrive at the same conclusion.

At a similar time, Dr. Semmelweis showed that when a midwife washed their hands in a solution before childbirth, the mortality rate of mothers decreased from 32% to zero. It was becoming clear that sanitation, hygiene, and cleanliness were some of the ways to reduce the spread of disease. Sterile consciousness that had been forgotten since the Greek and Roman times was being rediscovered.

It may seem logical today but in Dr. Semmelweis's time, studies such as these were ignored by a large portion of the medical profession because doctors and surgeons construed the ideas as insulting and offensive. Dr. Semmelweis was violently opposed and was eventually committed to an insane asylum against his will, where he was beaten by guards and eventually died of his wounds.

In 1880 the vaccine company Wellcome was established in England. This had the support and backing of the government and medical professions who still did not have any data to prove the effectiveness of the small pox vaccine. Wellcome was one of the leading vaccine manufacturers during the 20th century and would eventually merge with GSK in 1995.

The Tide of Change

A great tide of public opinion was beginning to go against compulsory vaccination laws and as a result, the anti-vaccination movement started gaining momentum. This led to a demonstration in the industrial town of Leicester in 1885. Stories were beginning to spread of fathers of families with a child who had died from receiving a vaccine were being imprisoned because they refused to allow another one of their children to be vaccinated.

People were becoming increasingly doubtful that the smallpox vaccine was protecting them from the disease. This was shown in the 1871-72 pandemic, despite the high systematic vaccination rate which had been placed upon the public. In the eighty years since their inception in 1796, they'd been shown as a disastrous failure, being compared with redundant medical procedures such as bloodletting and mercerisation. The Leicester demonstration was a culmination of the people not being listened to and the government's persistence in following a sunk cost fallacy (£20,000 had been invested in the smallpox vaccine by 1853).

The demonstration gained attention from both the rest of Europe and the USA and was attended by delegates from all over the UK. A procession two miles long marched through the town along with a crowd of up to 100,000 people holding banners such as "they that are whole need, not a physician." This showed that people of the time had an understanding of holistic principles. The conduct of the 100,000 people in attendance was exemplary to those who witnessed it, intending to bring fair and constitutional means to repel the laws.

The people of Leicester and their supporters had a plan that was also being backed by the scientific research of Dr. Semmelweis. Mr Councillor Butcher addressed the crowd by saying "A large and increasing portion of the public believed that the best way to get rid of smallpox and similar diseases was to use plenty of water, eat good food, live in light airy houses and see that the corporation kept the streets clean and drains in order."

This is a clear indication that the people of the time believed the successful solution was to improve sanitation standards, instead of following mass vaccinations. Mr. William Young then talked about the compulsory vaccination laws on our liberties, "that they are destructive of parental rights." People were expressing that they wanted to make their own decisions for both their health and the health of their children.

The demonstration was a huge success because the people had been able to make their feelings clear in a non-violent, articulate, and passionate way, against what they deemed were draconian measures encroaching on their civil liberty. Had the government put their time, money, and energy into dealing with the cause of the problem, namely cleaning up sanitation and taking Dr. Semmelweis science of hygiene on board sooner, the pseudoscience of the smallpox vaccine could have been discontinued by the end of the 19th Century.

The powers that be in Leicester continued to oppose the compulsory vaccination laws, so that as of 1885 onwards there were no more prosecutions for refusal. The smallpox vaccine had dropped from 95% to 5% of total births. The medical profession threatened residents that their decision would backfire and the town would suffer greatly from the disease, spreading like "wildfire on a prairie" and condemning people to death. However, both the leaders and the people of Leicester stuck to their decision and went ahead implementing changes to sanitation standards, hygiene, and isolating existing cases.

This later became known as the Leicester method. It involved an early detection of cases so that they could be quarantined in fever hospitals (separate units within hospitals) along with their families or housemates, while the house in question was thoroughly disinfected. This process resulted in the outbreak being successfully contained, even though the vaccination rates had dropped dramatically.

The success seen in Leicester meant that most towns across the country would go on to implement this method. In 1893 in Leicester, eight years after the demonstration, figures showed that the mortality rate in under ten-year-old children was 144 per million compared with Mold, a well- vaccinated town in Flintshire which had 3,614 per million. Leicester's smallpox numbers continued to drop year after year until the last major outbreak in 1904. There was only 1 case in 1906 and zero cases for the next four years.

Experts were beginning to take notice of this and started to question the efficacy of vaccines. Professor Crookshank wrote in 1889 "It is more probable that when, by means of notification and isolation, smallpox is kept under control, vaccination will disappear from practice and will retain only an historical interest." He believed the reason for the support of vaccines was due to enforced education by medical practitioners and that this flawed procedure would take a generation to be acknowledged as so.

Little credit was and is still given to Leicester for its part in the successful elimination of repetitive outbreaks of smallpox and the example it set in helping to eradicate the disease, even though the method would expand and be followed by the rest of England and the world. In a town with a population of a quarter of a million people, it was proven that pro vaccinators were wrong, by demonstrating that an unvaccinated population using the 'Leicester method' was less susceptible to smallpox than a 95% vaccinated population.

After the successful implementation of the Leicester method, smallpox outbreaks had become less virulent and the symptoms less lethal, even though fewer people were being vaccinated. Three main factors were the reason for this: hygiene, purification of water, and the introduction of sewers. Through the progressive advances in sanitation, the infrastructure of all diseases was on the decline.

This new understanding of sanitation prompted the construction of the London sewage system in 1859 which was a triumph of civil engineering. Wastewater was separated to provide clean water to the general public. The sewers in London, finished in 1880s were the first of their kind in the modern world and other cities around the world would all follow suit.

Leicester was an alternative drop of water in a sea of governmental support for vaccination programs by many nations. Punishments continued to be administered worldwide for those who decided not to vaccinate. People were sentenced to hard labour, fines, and imprisonment. Vaccinators would attend homes and work environments with police officers, using heavy-handed tactics. Those who still refused would be hauled to court and prosecuted.

In 1901, officers attended the American Tobacco Company where 350 women objected to compulsory vaccination, led by a woman called Florence Haskell. They attempted to make a stand by leaving the building but were held against their will and forced by the officers to be vaccinated as they struggled, screamed, and attempted to resist.

No one was exempt from these unjust rulings. A teacher in the state of Pennsylvania was threatened by a court that if she didn't receive a vaccination, she would be denied her right to teach. This overt blackmail, forcing her for her to comply was commonplace. Teachers and physicians were suspended until they permitted their pupils and patients to become vaccinated. In 1918 a solider refusing to be vaccinated was sentenced to 15 years in military prison.

There were numerous stories of people being forced against their will to either be vaccinated or face severe consequences. Their grounds for refusing were generally as a result of seeing loved ones hurt or killed by the vaccine, or seeing them still contracting the disease afterward. None of these reasons were taken seriously, as authorities continued to push towards absolute power over individuals.

There was a more sinister political ideology threatening the birthrights of civil liberties, which was being used in conjunction with the pro-vaccination movement of the early 20th century. Eugenics was a set of beliefs and practices which aimed to improve the genetic quality of the human population, typically by excluding people and groups judged to be inferior and promoting those who were judged to be superior.

Darwin's theory of natural selection was being used as a decree to enforce sterilisation (a medical procedure carried out to make a person infertile) of individuals deemed not worthy enough to reproduce. These practices started in the US, Nordic countries, and Nazi Germany. Hereditary health courts would sterilise those with conditions such as feeble-mindedness, schizophrenia, manic depression, epilepsy, genetic disorders, blindness and deafness.

This was considered to improve and enhance the human race by deleting defective genes from the collective gene pool. Eugenics believed that these people would go on to have defective and inferior children. Experts insisted that eugenics would help to reduce poverty, delinquency, and crime by eliminating these genes it outweighed the interest of the individual.

Supporters of this new branch of so-called 'science' were using the same kind of threatening and manipulative reasoning as the pro vaccinators. They insisted that if sterilisation was not implemented, thousands of children would be born with birth defects and that the public needed to be protected against this. They argued that sterilisation was for the domination of a superior race in the same way that vaccines were for our safety. The intention was to mould nature and society with biological technology.

By 1933 several countries had legal rights for sterilisation which could be forced upon anyone. Bar the Nazi regime the laws were implemented on a small scale however, 25,403 US citizens were sterilised in 1937, mostly in the state of California. The laws were considered a form of patriotism that enabled society to be safer and economically richer. These ideas of radical betterment were beginning to stretch further and further afield. They originated with prejudices against people with defects but would go on to discriminate against anyone, including creeds and ethnic minorities.

Absolute government power had taken away the personal liberties of individuals by forcing vaccines and sterilisation upon them. Eugenics was a science used without morality to be prejudiced against people for their creed, parentage, personality, intelligence, and situational circumstances. The outbreak and conclusion of the Second World War would lead eugenic ideology to contribute to the genocide of 6 million Jewish people. In the aftermath of the war, liberal democracy however, began to rise, and with it was the fall of eugenics as an accepted science or practice.

In 1948 which was the year compulsory vaccination ended in the UK, there were estimated 200-300 deaths as a direct result of the vaccine, compared with 1 death from smallpox during that time. In the previous 62 years since vaccination laws were abandoned in 1885, Leicester only had 53 deaths up until 1904 and only two in the following 40 years. Vaccinations for smallpox were declining nationally and so was the disease. From 1933-1946 there were only 28 deaths in a population of 40 million. In 1948 more people had died caused by the vaccination in one year than all the deaths from smallpox throughout the 20th Century.

The smallpox vaccine was removed in the late 20th century. The disease was proclaimed to have successfully eradicated single-handedly by the vaccine. Its chequered past of ineffectiveness and lethality to be forgotten and replaced with martyr status by pro vaccinators.

"Despite all the serious problems with its effectiveness, lack of evidence, it is still held up as the exemplary vaccine to promote vaccine faith today." This is a quote from dissolving illusions regarding the smallpox vaccine. All this information on the hidden past of vaccines can be found in this book.

Herd Immunity

When someone recovers from an infection such as measles, it engages their innate, cellular immune system and toll receptors. This is called whole cell immunity sometimes also known as memory immunity. This means the body has been through a complete process by identifying the infection, controlling the infection and then removing the infection. Innate antibodies are then used if exposed to the infection in the future to stop re-infection and also stop person to person spread, which is why it's also known as memory immunity. Whole cell immunity does not happen when we are inoculated with vaccines because our bodies go through a shorter process to that of whole cell immunity. The only similar aspect is that medically induced antibodies are released, which is the end process of whole cell immunity.

Imagine taking your car for an MOT, the mechanic assesses what changes need to happen for you your car to pass it's MOT and be road worthy. In this analogy this would be whole cell immunity; making your car and other road users safe. However, imagine the mechanic may or may not check your car but still gave you an MOT certificate. This represents medically induced antibodies where the car is possibly a safety hazard and a risk to you and other drivers. The analogy isn't perfect however this alludes to a complex process in the body compared with the vaccine response.

It is completely natural for our bodies to become sick every once in a while. A good example of this is when a dog is ill they will eat grass, sit in the shade, and sometimes vomit up the grass. Nobody tells the dog to do this but they follow this instinctively when they feel unwell. We get infectious diseases for many reasons but one is that our bodies need to go through a detoxification process. The medical model of suppressing the symptoms of infections through vaccines goes against nature and the way that our bodies intuitively heal themselves.

If you have a cold, what does your body do? Mucus membranes are stimulated to secrete fluid, which make our sinuses become runny. What about if we had a belly ache? We might need to vomit or excrete toxins. What about an infection? More than likely we will experience a fever to assist the T cells to kill and remove the antigens which are then cleared up by antibodies. These processes are all normal functions that occur in our immune systems and they happen automatically when we are healthy.

The term "herd immunity" was originally coined in the 1930s. Researchers realised that the spread of measles was declining in areas where the rate of infection of the population had reached 50-60% of people that had been infected and successfully recovered (whole cell immunity). Therefore stopping person to person spread and also protecting others that had not yet been infected. The R figure (the rate at which the infection spreads), went from 2.2 to under 1. This means that on average one infected person will infect 2.2 people and so the infection spreads, as opposed to an R figure less than 1 means that every infected person will, on average, infect zero to 1 person, leading to the suppression of the infection.

These statistics show if children were allowed to build up a natural immunity to infections such as measles, occasional measles outbreaks would occur but it would be controllable as the R figure would remain low because of herd immunity (percentage of population with whole cell/memory immunity/stopping person to person spread). When the measles vaccine was introduced in 1963 the term herd immunity was used by vaccine manufacturers to mean not whole cell/memory immunity, but instead to describe the percentage of the population that had been vaccinated. In the new herd immunity the percentage went from 50-60% (actual herd immunity) to 95% (5% population were not vaccinated because they were exempt) of children needed for herd immunity. Basically 95% of children were needed to be vaccinated to achieve herd immunity.

It has been suggested that the reason why herd immunity percentage was increased from whole cell immunity of 50-60% to 95% with a vaccine, was because vaccines may protect against a virus, but medically induced antibodies do not stop person to person spread compared with whole cell immunity.

With certain vaccines a person can still contract the particular infection related to the vaccine, called the antigen sin. This is when a vaccine stimulates the immune system to produce antibodies but if the vaccine does not confer immunity to the infection and the person becomes infected, the immune system does not react because antibodies are present. Therefore; the immune system is tricked into thinking the infection is under control, turning a more likely non-life threatening infection, in a healthy person, to a potentially life threatening situation.

Instead of implementing immunisation programs, if the population was allowed build up whole cell immunity (herd immunity) to these infections, there would be small clusters of outbreaks but their spread would be limited by the large amount of people that confer whole cell immunity, therefore limiting person to person spread. Leaving the question is it better to let nature take its course and allow people to develop whole cell immunity in 50-60% of the population? Or to use mass inoculations that requires 95% participation to suppress an infection?

As we already discussed, if the population was allowed to reach the level needed for herd immunity then the outbreaks would be minimal and those exposed would be creating real immunity to infections in the way that nature intended. Eradication of measles through vaccines is impossible otherwise it would already have happened. Not everyone who is vaccinated becomes immune which is why every two to three years we will see outbreaks of measles regardless of the numbers vaccinated.

Are vaccinations for you?

Making an informed decision is our responsibility and to do so we need to take an active role in understanding how the body works so that we can decide if vaccines are for us or not. Seek out medical professionals with a non-judgmental view on vaccines. We are led to believe vaccines are both necessary and safe offering total protection, but this isn't true, vaccines, like most drugs, come with side effects and need to be taken case by case to ensure they necessary and safe.

My suggestion is to fully discuss the possible side effects with your practitioner and weigh up the benefits and risks before proceeding. It's important to understand that you are injecting foreign matter into a human being to avoid an infection, with a small risk of severe side effects that could result in long term disability. Understanding these risks will help you make that trade-off decision.

My advice is that if you are considering vaccinations, schedule them carefully and spread them out over a longer period. This can give you peace of mind that one vaccine does not interact with another vaccine's side effects.

There are laboratory blood tests called tilter tests that can check if certain antibodies are already present in the bloodstream for bacteria and infections. This will reveal if a person is already immune to a certain virus. They are available for most infections and can help you make the best decision for both you and your loved ones. For example, if someone has already been exposed to the chickenpox virus but never developed symptoms, they may have an adequate antibody level and therefore this would suggest a vaccination in this instance, would be unnecessary.

We need to return to understanding the importance of a healthy diet, exercise, and emotional health.

When we are healthy, partake in regular exercise, eat wholesome foods, drink purified water and receive plenty of regular sleep, we are less likely to be susceptible to a) serious infections and b) if we do, our immune systems will be able to effectively fight the infection until full recovery is achieved. Research has shown that a child who exercises regularly has a higher white blood cell count than a child who does not.

History has shown us that the way we live our lives is the biggest factor in our health and wellbeing. These factors include receiving vital vitamins and minerals in our diet, making healthy changes to our living environment, and reducing the consumption of agricultural poisons sprayed on our crops. Refined sugars, white flour, alcohol, tobacco, and antibiotics can all contribute to raising inflammatory levels within the body, which results in disease.

History repeats itself

Pro vaccine lobby groups are convinced that they have the scientific evidence and there is no need to debate the effectiveness and safety of vaccines, when in fact the scientific evidence is conflicted. They state 'in a propaganda style' that the anti-vaccine movement is unscientific when in fact the people I've met that question the safety of vaccines, just want to be free to make their own health choices. It is hard to debate with an opponent that ignores, and covers up the other side's argument.

Science is a theory that is tested extensively and accurately, after which observations are made as to the possible different outcomes. These theories are then tested for their robustness and over time the weight of evidence supports and proves and disproves them. This is an infinite cycle of reflection and refining of the sciences, to a continually changing theory. As time goes forward and we progress further, we simply have more effective ways to test our current paradigm theories.

Science unfortunately is being used as a political tool used by pro-vaccinators to stifle the vaccine debate.

The anti-vaccine debate is valid scientifically, morally, and justly. I believe that if there was a level playing field when debating the effectiveness of vaccines, there is no doubt in my mind that the scientific case for vaccines would lack robustness compared with the research on whole cell immunity performed in the early 20th century.

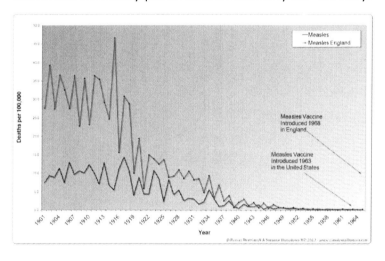

Graph showing measles was declining long before the vaccine.

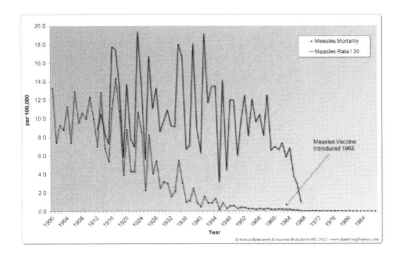

The bottom line in the graph shows the mortality rate of Measles was declining long before the vaccine was developed.

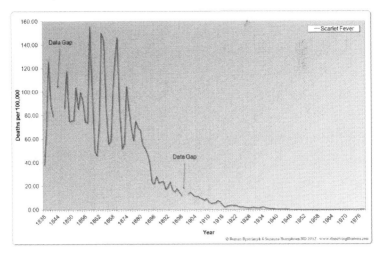

This graph shows the mortality rate of Scarlett fever from 1838-1976. There was a vaccine for Scarlet fever but it wasn't widely used because it was even more lethal than the smallpox vaccine. Here we can see even in spite of the vaccine not being widely used, Scarlet Fever still declined.

The elephant in the room is that all infections were on the decline long before vaccines were introduced. The sanitation revolution which began in the mid-19th Century is strong evidence to suggest this was the reason that brought a halt to the spread of a great number of infections and diseases, causing them to decline. City sewage works were created to separate waste from drinking water, hygiene vastly improved, labour laws were introduced. Innovations such as electricity, refrigeration, transportation and flushable toilets were invented to improve the quality of living and health.

It was clear from my research that the largest decline in cases of smallpox happened at the turn of the 20th Century when isolation techniques and sanitation were adopted seriously. The smallpox vaccine was in my view a failure, worse than dud; it killed more people than it saved of smallpox during the 20th century and the same is likely the 19th Century. One must ask the question, if smallpox was eradicated by a vaccine, why has measles or other flu like viruses not been eradicated by their vaccine?

In infections such as measles and other childhood illnesses, the mortality rate was declining long before their particular vaccine arrived. No vaccine was ever produced for typhus, typhoid or cholera and many others, but they declined too, which makes the sanitation argument even stronger.

During the Covid 19 lockdown in the spring of 2020, every time I opened a newspaper, there was an article reporting a study of the benefits of vaccines. In one study they proclaimed 'vaccine prevents dementia', when I read the article there was merely a causal link, which actually means that it could have been lifestyle or any other reason, as much as it could have been the effect of the vaccine. Yet that was what got the headline.

The health and social care, sectary of state at the time Matt Hancock had claimed that millions of doses of the Oxford vaccine, which is being developed at the University of Oxford, are being prepared for distribution even before the vaccine has received an emergency license. The vaccine has only been tested on the young and healthy so far and the people that are considered to be most in need, no tests have been done, but they are still talking up the Oxford vaccine as the only 'saviour' to return our lives to normal.

I believe a focus on developing a treatment plan that reduces the mortality rate for Covid 19, would be more effective than a flu vaccine, which will need to be administered and redesigned annually; therefore, the virus spreading would be less of problem. Contracting the virus could be good for us because this would build memory immunity that could provide cross immunity to other cold and flu viruses. We would then be less susceptible to the next virus outbreak. These are simple, natural principles that our ancestors intuitively knew, so when did getting sick become this thing to avoid at all cost?

Getting sick once in a while is important for your body to naturally detox and clear itself out. We have to get away from this fear of others and accept that we spread germs like we have spread ideas to each other since the beginning of mankind. The more we allow fear of a flu virus of short duration to proliferate, the more likely we'll see xenophobic behaviours and prejudice of others in our communities.

Artificial protection against infections through vaccines could do us more harm than good in the long run. When explorers from Europe in the 16th Century discovered the Americas they brought with them the diseases that circulated Europe such as smallpox. The indigenous population were wiped out as their immune systems had no memory immunity to protect them from these new diseases that Europeans were hardened to. Therefore consider that you could walk around in a space suit for a number of years but once you come out of the space suit, you will be more at risk from new infection than otherwise.

In the UK vaccines are still optional. You can choose to decline them. However, in countries such as the US and Australia, laws are being set in motion to make them compulsory. Pressure is being applied to parents; they are told that if they do not consent to vaccines, their children will be excluded from school, which is blackmail. This is also illogical reasoning, if vaccines were as effective as we are being told then children who did receive the vaccine would not be at any risk from the few that do not partake. These are the same tactics of intimidation that were used in the first wave of compulsory vaccination laws, that the unvaccinated are a threat to the vaccinated.

In an industry that is growing year by year, (for example $10 billion has been invested by the Gates Foundation from 2010 to 2020) lobby groups are pushing for "the evolution of healthy people in 2020". They propose to have a 95% vaccination rate in all age groups for the flu shot and an 80% vaccination rate of all the other vaccines. There are bills of rights in the USA ready to implement so that vaccines become compulsory, therefore removing citizens' right to choose.

One day most of us will need some kind of medical intervention especially as we continue to age. I believe in these types of intervention where appropriate, but I have trouble understanding how it is possible to force vaccinations onto people, when the past of vaccines is so dubious. I believe this is immoral and it would be a crime against humanity if our choice is taken away.

I am not denying that vaccines are effective at suppressing certain infections; however I do question their effectiveness in eradicating smallpox and believe the claim is exaggerated. I would be more likely to accept a vaccine if older versions were to be redesigned by removing heavy metals and other toxic chemicals. I'd like scientists to explore homeopathic remedies or variolation techniques verses vaccines. Do we need such heavy doses to confer immunity? Could a smaller micro dose be just as effective, therefore reducing the risks?

I also want to make clear that I am not anti-vaccine. I am in fact, pro-choice. I am someone who wants to have all the risks laid out transparently, such as what the vaccines contain and what their short and long term risk is to my health. I would like people to be able to have a discussion where we can challenge the current status quo, without accusation, implying that a person with these views is irresponsible with their own life and they are risking others people's lives by even considering to not to be immunised. The fear and guilt projection by the pro-vaccination movement is a paradox because I feel they are the ones being irresponsible and risking lives by not acknowledging these concerns.

The pro-vaccine movement and their lobby groups could turn out to be modern-day snake oil salesman. They are preaching the benefits of vaccines without considering their risks and long term implications and they are pressurising governments to make them more inclusive than ever. At least snake oil salesman and their bogus products were in some cases harmless. Vaccines however, are not harmless and have considerable risks. The pro-vaccine movement has taken their belief structure beyond science and it borders on fanatical religious indoctrination. When vaccines do not live up to their promises, the blame is always placed upon the unvaccinated, or that more doses are required for the vaccines to be effective.

So, the next time Bill Gates tells us that people in poorer economic countries are at risk because they have not received their vaccines, please consider that the reason they may become sick is not because they haven't had a vaccine. It's equally plausible they become sick because of their living conditions. These are more of a risk to them in causing a disease, similar to that of our ancestors in the 19th century. Perhaps Bill Gates' $10 billion could be used instead for sustainable farming, better nutrition, and sanitation of poorer nations to make a far bigger impact than a jab in the arm.

Kudos to Mark Zuckerberg when he protected free speech by resisting pressure to remove posts of people's concerns regarding vaccines on Facebook because he said it's fair to question their effectiveness or express doubts about how they are administered. "If someone is pointing out a case where a vaccine caused harm or that they are worried about them, it is a difficult thing from my perspective, to say 'you shouldn't be allowed to express that at all'".

This is written as an alternative view to vaccines that isn't always reported, explaining the lesser known history, busting the myth that they were the reason for life expectancy to increase, to reveal a hidden, uglier truth. You might be wondering why I've dedicated a whole chapter to vaccines. Well the reason is that all the while that we focus on the use of vaccines in our modern healthcare system, the focus is taken away from preventive lifestyle modifications and mindset management, that are equal if not more important than vaccines in health matters. We promote vaccines as total protection, and in doing so, people being vaccinated risk neglecting lifestyle changes as a result.

Vaccines are celebrated as transforming our fight against disease but I hope this chapter puts those claims into perspective. People were less likely to die of killer diseases at the beginning of the 20th Century than decades earlier because of improvements to sanitation which are generally claimed to be as a result of vaccines by modern medicine. However most vaccines were introduced many years later, therefore I question do they deserve the credit modern medicine places upon them? Instead as stated in dissolving illusions, "sunshine, fresh air, wholesome foods, exercise, rest, and hygiene proved to be far more effective than all the vaccines in existence".

Chapter 3: Covid-19

"It is becoming more and more obvious that it is not starvation, it is not microbes, it is not cancer, but man himself who is his greatest danger: because he has no adequate protection against psychic epidemics, which are infinitely more devastating in their effect than the greatest natural catastrophes."

Carl Jung

Part I: Stay Home, Protect the NHS, Save Lives (and discard your common sense)

Governments and large institutions shape our world with rules and regulations which they say protect us from harm and potential danger, but often they use fear to gain compliance. When a person succumbs to this fear, they surrender their decision making to an outside source, instead of trusting their instincts. Often the information we are given is incorrect or even worse than that, those in power exploit and control their position, covering up their incompetence, shifting blame and even worse, knowingly stand to gain from decisions that are not in the general public's interests.

The freedom our past generations fought for and preserved is being dramatically altered in the blink of an eye, due to our improvised response to a novel flu strain. The boundary between personal freedom and state power has shifted and is ushering in a new era of censoring, surveillance, and unthinkable restrictions, which will still be in place long after this crisis is over. Welcome to the 'new normal'.

In the spring of 2020, the country was placed under house arrest in the hope of suppressing a virus that was already in the mitigation phase (impossible to eradicate). This means there was no effective way of containing the virus because the horse had already bolted. Guided by imperfect models and caveat laden data, we were taken on an extraordinary journey. This chapter will look into the response of both the UK government and countries from all over the world in more depth and ask if their actions were justified.

The UK was one of the worst affected countries not only in Europe but in the world due to the reactionary nature of the UK government's response. However, 90% of the deaths from Covid 19 are people over 60 years of age. The mortality rate average age is between, 80-88 which is higher than the UK life expectancy. If you are young and healthy without any underlying health conditions, you are more likely to die in a car accident than from Covid 19. If you are under the age of 16 you are more likely to be hit by lightning than die from Covid 19. When we consider these figures against the government's response do they seem proportionate? (It's ok if you're scratching your head at the moment; you're not the only one).

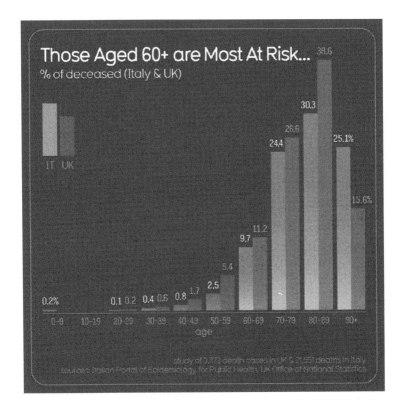

Those Aged 60+ are Most At Risk...
% of deceased (Italy & UK)

IT UK

0.2%   0.1 0.2   0.4 0.6   0.8   1.7   2.5   5.4   9.7   11.2   24.4   26.6   30.3   38.6   25.1%   15.6%

0-9   10-19   20-29   30-39   40-49   50-59   60-69   70-79   80-89   90+
age

study of 3,373 death cases in UK & 21,551 deaths in Italy
sources: Italian Portal of Epidemiology for Public Health, UK Office of National Statistics

Graph showing the elderly (over 60 years of age) being the most at risk from this virus. You would struggle to find a graph of any given year that looks dissimilar to this graph showing the mortality rate for any reason.

Corona viruses were first discovered in 1965 when scientists identified the first human corona virus associated with the common cold. The corona virus family is named because of their "crown-like" appearance in their molecular structure. There currently 36 different strains, 3 of which are highly common and have been present for sixty years. More recently we have seen severe acute respiratory syndrome (SARS), Middle Eastern respiratory syndrome (MERS) and now severe acute respiratory syndrome-corona virus -2 (Covid 19.)

The CDC estimates that 35% of people who have been infected with Covid 19 will be asymptomatic and estimates the mortality rate is 0.26%. From the very beginning, it was clear the elderly and those with underlying health conditions like COPD, heart disease, cancer, obesity, and diabetes were most at risk. It takes little common sense to work out these stats would stand for any cold or flu virus, the only extraordinary aspect of these figures is they are being highlighted to us.

Enter the Dragon

As early as November 2019 in the Chinese city of Wuhan, a new flu strain called SARS-CoV-2 was discovered. It was renamed in March by The World Health Organisation (WHO) and became more commonly known as Covid 19. It is believed that the virus originated from China's wild animal trade, specifically from wet markets known for their live exotic animals and meat, sold in close proximity together. It is thought that cross-contamination could have happened which may have resulted in the spread of the virus to humans.

In late December, a doctor in the city of Wuhan named Dr Li Wenliang discovered there was a group of people with similar symptoms of an unknown illness. He tried to warn fellow clinicians but was subsequently arrested for spreading rumours and forced to agree to stop speaking out. He returned to work, where sadly he contracted Covid 19 and died as a result.

In early January Professor Zhang Yongzhen, a scientist in Shanghai had made an extraordinary breakthrough by sequencing the genome of the Covid 19. He immediately reported his findings to China's National Health Commission and recommended an introduction of disease control measures. The Communist Party of China (CCP) decided not to take any action, and six days later Professor Zhang published the data on two open-source sites for scientists all around the world to access. The next day his lab was shut down and has not reopened since.

Two nurses who volunteered in Wuhan published a letter in the Lancet calling for international assistance but this was quickly retracted by the authorities who denied acknowledgement of human to human transmissions, even after warnings by Taiwanese scientists. They refused to cooperate with the WHO in the early stages of studying Covid 19, leaving other countries to guess the nature of the threat.

The Wuhan seafood wholesale markets were a cause for concern as there was a cluster of 24 people infected with pneumonia with no clear cause, dating back to early December. One of the first people to be struck down with the infection was the wife of a market trader.

The first death was on the 10th of January, and on the 23rd of January, a lockdown in Wuhan was put into place. Videos on social media showed the people of Wuhan were prevented from leaving their home, by welding their doors closed.

It appeared that the CCP was more interested in covering up the situation than helping the international community. Instead of praising the brave scientists, doctors, and nurses for their efforts, they censored them in an attempt to control and conceal the virus. Had they acted promptly when Dr Li Wenliang warned of the infection in December and fully cooperated with WHO regulations putting an immediate travel ban in place, the virus may have been successfully contained in Wuhan.

China was embarking on a state-controlled campaign of relentless misinformation and secrecy. They were showing disdain for human rights by imposing draconian measures. Their refusal to act responsibly within their own country resulted in a huge number of unnecessary global deaths. They took huge political risks with their heavy-handed, ultra-nationalist approach, the breaking of treaties and threatening anyone who spoke out against them.

China has a track record of foul play, as places such as Taiwan and Hong Kong can attest. It would appear China's influence over the WHO was so great that they would not recognize Taiwan's Covid 19 figures because China did not class Taiwan as an independent state.

Another embarrassing moment in late March happened, when Bruce Aylward, a senior WHO adviser, was unable to respond to a question from a Hong Kong-based journalist concerning Taiwan independence.

China used the distraction of the Covid 19 outbreak to establish power enforcements over Hong Kong as they made sweeping plans to strip the island off the southern coast of China of its democratic freedoms. Chris Patten, the last governor of Hong Kong said this was a comprehensive assault on the fundamental freedoms agreed in Sino-British joint declaration.

Enter the WHO

The WHO is not the sixties band who sang "My Generation", although they would probably be more useful than the World Health Organization. The WHO was set up in 1954 after the Second World War as part of the United Nations, by a group of international politicians led by Winston Churchill. They were supposed to be the cream of the scientific community, who pooled together their talents and expertise for the greater good. They aimed to discover the most up to date solutions on health matters and to coordinate global responses while at the same time remaining impartial.

Their handling of the Covid 19 pandemic was shocking, to say the least. Their lack of impartiality and inability to criticize China has forced many people in the west to question the role of the WHO and if they can be trusted to coordinate global responses in future. The Japanese

Deputy Prime Minister, Tara Aso said that the WHO had grown far too close to China. Indeed he suggested it should change its name to the "Chinese Health Organisation".

After the SARS outbreak in 2007 the WHO introduced new International Health Regulations requiring countries to notify them within 24 hours, of all events that may constitute a public health emergency of international concern within their territory. Afterwards, continued accurate updates including test numbers, case numbers, and deaths were required. China failed to comply with these regulations.

The facts are that China had an unknown pneumonia epidemic they were aware of but they knowingly did not to release data to the WHO. The WHO failed to challenge the lack of data resulting in a failure to warn the rest of the world sooner. Governments around the world rely on the WHO as the most authoritative source of information on infectious diseases.

Taiwan warned the WHO in late December that there was evidence of person to person transmission but this was denied by China. The WHO ignored Taiwan's advice and stayed close to China's official line, even as the situation worsened. The WHO would go on to tweet on the 14th of January, "there was no evidence of human to human transmission", even though there was evidence.

However just a week later, The Head of the WHO, Tedros Adhanom, praised China's response to the epidemic as exemplary. He said that Chinese officials had shown commitment in combating the transmission of the virus and demonstrated cooperation with other countries to stem its global spread. "Its actions actually helped prevent the spread of Covid 19 to other countries," he said. China had been taking extraordinary measures in the face of what was an extraordinary challenge.

These examples show the influence China had over the WHO. Slowly, they stepped up its warnings and advice, finally declaring a global public health emergency on 30th January. However, their lack of impartiality, reluctance to act and challenge China is questionable.

Enter Italy

Initially, Italy was the country worse hit by the virus in Europe. By the 7th of March, they had an epicentre in the region of Lombardy which was beginning to overwhelm the health service. On this same day, Italy was due to play Ireland in the six nations but it was cancelled because of the threat of Covid 19. This was to be the start of cancellations of sport and mass gatherings across most of Europe.

Football and other sports continued for another few days but on Friday 13th March the majority of sports except for rugby league had cancelled schedules with reviews to commence again in April. For Italy to have an epicentre by 7th March, shows how long the virus had been present in the country. If you think about it for a moment, how long did it take for London to become the epicentre? It probably took another month or so.

This is the start of the scientific bias that created an unrealistic hype surrounding the virus. The Covid 19 numbers were only being measured on people who needed medical intervention and those who unfortunately died and not those who presented symptoms. Testing numbers were not high enough to gather meaningful data on total infections therefore the mortality rate was inflated beyond reality.

On 9th March Italy imposed a nation-wide lockdown believed to be the largest suppression of constitutional rights by any western democratic country in peacetime. Italy had seen what had happened in China and believed that following a similar lockdown was the best practice. However, as we know, China's motive for the lockdown was based on covering up and concealing the virus and its origins, which was not in the best interests of their citizens and the world. The UK would be next to implement this drastic measure, closely followed by the rest of Europe.

Enter the Bulldog (minus the spirit)

Up until 16th March, the people of Britain were instructed to wash their hands to the tune of happy birthday and to continue on with their lives as usual. If someone became ill or showed any symptoms of Covid 19 they were advised to self-isolate for 7 days. Anyone who had been in close proximity to them was advised to do the same for 14 days. We were practising the Leicester model to identify and isolate. The government was following the policy of herd immunity, a long term strategy, which over time would stop person to person transmission, therefore reducing the R figure of future waves.

News agencies were clear that people over a certain age with underlying health conditions were most at risk and those that were healthy, were more likely to be less affected. The advice of receiving adequate sunshine, vitamins, and exercise was still being promoted, as long as people took the recommended precautions. This empowered individuals to help themselves by making good health choices. This common-sense approach was and could have worked well but the message was about to change drastically.

On the 16th March, Professor Neil Ferguson from Imperial College London (ICL) gave a presentation to the Government predicting that half a million people would die if a lockdown was not implemented. This is the part of the story where we entered a unique time, where unprecedented decisions were made that have never been seen before in modern history, but are now seen as the 'new normal'.

Within a week the UK entered a lockdown and like dominos most European countries would follow suit shortly afterwards. When the Swedish epidemiologist, Anders Tegnell, was questioned about Sweden's approach to rejecting a lockdown, he said they (Sweden) were following empirical evidence, that nationwide lockdowns had never been attempted and "it was the rest of the world that was performing an experiment."

Stay Home

On the 23rd March draconian measures had been implemented, laws were changed so that businesses were forced to shut, nonessential workers were told to stay at home, only key workers were allowed to work and travel and schools were closed nationally. Children still went to school in wartime. We had entered a police state where it was now a crime to swim in the sea, sunbathe in a public park or visit anyone outside your household, as it was considered to be risking lives (no measure was given to how many lives our compliance would save). The virus at this point had already peaked meaning that cases were already declining.

We were being warned of an invisible virus that was vastly different from seasonal flu and could kill any age group. The 'killer virus' was now a mental image that was being projected on to us whenever we switched on the news, read a paper, or on adverts. Celebrities were enlisted to help reinforce the message to stay at home but where had all the messaging gone about good hygiene, sunlight, and keeping healthy?

Journalists paraphrased politicians from the daily briefing, writing that the virus did not discriminate. We were told that we were all at risk and that no one was safe. An indiscriminate lockdown was put in place for all.

News agencies were becoming extremely unrealistic, dramatizing events and projecting all ages and health statuses, suggesting there was a high chance they could die from this 'killer virus'. It was shameful journalism that should be sanctioned. You Tube content with alternative views were censored because this did not fit with the government narrative, being that the virus was lethal to anyone and we should be afraid. This misinformation by media outlets caused a huge amount of unnecessary fear and hysteria, which in my opinion needs to be held accountable.

For this reason I shun news that is reported in a headline grabbing way. They knowingly take peoples comments out of context to twist them to create a narrative, which paints them as the villain or lacking virtues. It is a dehumanizing process based on manipulation and inauthentic reporting of daily occurrences to mass audiences.

The government felt they needed full compliance with the lockdown to enable them to control the virus but they had no control over those posting on social media and video platforms. The CEO of YouTube, Susan Wojcicki announced measures to remove videos "medically unsubstantiated", including anything which went against WHO guidelines. The information deemed good advice was being measured by an organisation that we already mentioned lacked impartially and integrity.

Those who held alternative views were censored or marginalized with labelled stereotypes. These events were landmarks in all our lives and people were restricted from expressing themselves, debating the subject, or questioning why we were all being locked up. We were force-fed government slogans and woke up every morning to what felt like Groundhog Day. It is not difficult to see why many of the public felt sceptical, uncertain, and isolated.

Peter Ebdon, a snooker player, was asked his opinion regarding the virus on a Radio Five Live show. He said that he "felt building herd immunity" could be more beneficial in the longer term for the collective than a lockdown. He finished his interview by saying, "in my honest opinion we are facing the greatest psychological operation in history."

Whether you agree or disagree with Peter is irrelevant. He had an opposing view which was labelled by most newspapers as a conspiracy theory and they claimed the BBC was wrong to allow him to express his view. Polarizing these views stifles a healthy debate. When did it become illegal to have an opinion?

Democracy is built on freedom of speech. People should be allowed to express themselves and make up their own minds. If you censor debate all you do is drive the ideas underground where they cannot be seen, valued, or challenged. People need to be able to openly express their ideas to honour their freedom of speech and to allow them to be challenged.

One of the greatest inventions of the 20th century was the World Wide Web, a nervous system for the planet, given to us by Sir Tim Berners-Lee. He decided the internet should be free to use, which was a benevolent gesture in a world driven by profit. To censor the internet is a slippery slope that in time could erode liberal democracies. To quote Aldous Huxley, "the perfect dictatorship would have the appearance of democracy, but would basically be a prison without walls."

Enter Sunshine (staying at home costs lives)

The advice of receiving regular sunshine, vitamins, and exercise was dropped for the government's single-minded approach. Nothing else mattered except reducing the spread of the virus. The basic rights of individuals were replaced by rules of the state claiming to protect and make healthy choices for us. We were disempowered from making our own decisions regarding our health and well-being.

Sunlight is known to be a germicidal and there is growing evidence that it can kill viruses. Science from the sixties showed that outdoor air is a natural disinfectant with an ability to kill flu viruses and protect against viral transmission. It is believed that UV rays damage the DNA and RNA structure of a virus by degrading the fatty protein, outer casing. When you stay at home indoors, it is far easier to catch a respiratory infection than if you are outside, especially with poor ventilation or if your home or office is serviced by air conditioning units.

Members within the government such as Matt Hancock, accused people of sunbathing in parks as "putting others lives at risk." The empirical evidence however is not supported by forcing people to stay indoors; therefore, preventing them from receiving vitamin D, which scientific evidence supports is good for us.

Following the Science

'Following the science' has been the UK government's response to answer difficult questions since the beginning of the outbreak. However, it is not clear what science they are following, as the scientific community was divided much like the population. We have heard experts argue over the Sweden model, the use of ventilators, if wearing a mask is effective protection, and whether children are at risk or not.

Almost every day we are bombarded with a new study on how the infection spreads: it is airborne/ it is on surfaces, you are safe outside/you're at risk inside. It will take years before the virus's dynamics of transmission have been fully agreed upon. Therefore, if the scientific community cannot agree amongst themselves, whose science is the government following?

The measures taken by the UK government and their effectiveness are highly debatable, splitting public support; it seemed that people were either for or against the lockdown. Those who wanted stringent restrictions wanted them to be enforced more tightly and for a longer period. Others wanted fewer restrictions and for them to be lifted sooner. How much of the public support for tighter restrictions were due to the reporting of the virus being deadlier than in reality and the fear mongering that was spread by the government and news outlets?

It was Albert Einstein who said, "The only source of knowledge is experience." In our current world using 'following the science' as a dogma, we are lacking the value of our experience. Science is best when balanced with our experiences. 'Following the science' is in danger of becoming an esoteric practice to produce interventional gimmicks (nationwide lockdowns), while ignoring individual circumstances, holistic principles, and natural phenomena.

Enter SAGE

The Scientific Advisory Group for Emergencies (SAGE) is the 'committee' that guided government ministers to make their decisions. Not to be confused with a sage of the past; someone or something who is wise or exhibits signs of wisdom and intelligence.

Within SAGE is the government's fall guy, Professor Neil Ferguson. As mentioned earlier his modelling (which was never peer reviewed at the time) convinced the government that, according to his research 500,000 people would die if a nationwide lockdown was not implemented. The government performed an about turn in favour of a Chinese/Italian style lockdown.

Once the modelling had been released, computer programmers carried out tests which showed the modelling was highly inaccurate. The code was outdated, incoherent, and completely unreliable. As a team from Edinburgh University found out when they received two different results, when using the same code, they claimed "if we attempt two identical runs, only varying in that the second should use the network file produced by the first, the results are quite different."

The predictions made by the modelling were proved to be based on false assumptions such as the virus mortality rate being ten times higher than in reality. It seemed that embarrassing inaccuracies were nothing new to Professor Neil's work. In the foot and mouth outbreak of 2001, he advised the infected cattle to be culled but also those from nearby farms, even if there was no outbreak or signs of the disease. This led to 6 million cattle being slaughtered, an action that other epidemiologists argued was unnecessary.

In 2002, he also predicted that 136,000 people would die from Mad Cow Disease but the actual death total was only 200. In 2005 he told the Guardian that 200 million would die from bird flu. The final death toll was just over 400 people. Finally, he proclaimed that swine flu would kill 65,000 people but the total UK deaths were approximately 460. It begs the question as to why the government sought the advice of Professor Ferguson in the first place before mothballing our multitrillion pound economy and plunging millions of people into poverty and hardship.

They put a lot of faith in someone who did not have a successful track record. Journalists described his work as crystal ball modelling. If his role was performance-related, he would have been sacked a long time ago. This was his eventual fate but not as a result of criticisms of his inability to predict epidemiological events, Ferguson was in fact forced to resign after flouting his own lockdown recommendations, when he was visited by a woman from another household. His defence was that he thought he was immune because he had already had the virus.

This left everyone confused as to the dynamics of the virus and the rules. If a person had the virus and recovered, were they exempt from the rules because they would be immune? By following Fergusons' scientific advice, the government had too many rules based on assumptions that created holes, and every time they tried to plug the next hole, the problem (holes) had multiplied. They had chosen a complex strategy when Ockham razor would have been enough (the simplest answer with the least amount of assumptions is often the most effective and correct answer).

In contrast, there was modelling available from the University of Oxford that had conflicting figures to Ferguson's prediction. These would turn out to be much more accurate. On 14th March, Nobel Prize winner Michael Levitt at Stanford University predicted that the UK would lose about 50,000 lives. He wrote to the UK government's advisors and Ferguson telling them that his modelling of the mortality rate was overestimated by 10-12 times. Later he would say he thought the lockdown measures saved no lives, "I think lockdown will cause much, much more damage than the deaths saved."

Professor Levitt won his Nobel Prize in chemistry, has no background in epidemiology. However, he assessed the initial outbreak in China and used the data from the Cruise ship the "Diamond Princess" to make predictions on the virus. How could someone with no background in epidemiology, predict far more accurate results than a professor from ICL leading independent research? He said, "The problem with epidemiologists is that they feel their job is to frighten people into lockdown. So they say 'there's going to be a million deaths' and when there are only 25,000 they say 'it's good you listened to my advice.'"

Considering the risks the government were prepared to take on Ferguson's modelling, that did not take into account, for example, economic consequences, would it not have been wise to seek the advice of economists and mental health experts? Or at least have those experts' privy to SAGE meetings and decision making?

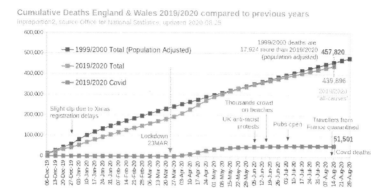

Graph showing similar mortality rate (top lines) this year with a previous year and no change to Covid 19 trajectory (bottom line) despite human interactions.

Enter Sweden

By the end of March 2020, most of the developed world had some form of arbitrary lockdown in place in an attempt to contain Covid 19. Sweden, however, had not changed course. Did they know something we didn't? Surrounding countries predicted Sweden's death toll from the virus would exceed more than any other country.

While the rest of the western world was pursuing an ill-fated scramble to try and contain the virus, Sweden adopted a different approach by continuing with empirical evidence to mitigate the virus. Moderate

129

measures were embraced in the hope of shielding the vulnerable and allowing healthy people to acquire the virus. Anders Bjorkman a professor of infectious diseases in Stockholm said, "The virus a little more active in younger people is not a big harm and you develop herd immunity."

Instead of a lockdown they kept shops and restaurants open (with guidance) and asked the nation to use their judgment. Already a high amount of trust existed between the people and the government and this demonstrated the relationship between them. The Swedes offered transparent advice and treated their citizens like adults, empowering them to make the best decision for them.

This came with much criticism early on from those outside Sweden. People were conflicted with their decision making, as there was an increase in people dying in the short term. Why were they not doing anything about this? The pressure was also coming internally and a petition was signed by 2000 Swedish doctors asking for more stringent measures to be put in place.

When questioned on their approach, Swedish Professor Johan Giesecke, the first Chief Scientist of the European Centre for Disease Prevention and Control, said that the virus amounted to a "tsunami of usually quite mild diseases" that would wash over Europe regardless of the lockdown, with at least half of the population becoming infected. Public health policy choices by individual countries would over time, have little impact on the number of deaths but the cost of the lockdown would far exceed those of a targeted strategy aimed at protecting the most vulnerable.

Sweden had the courage in their convictions to maintain the course they felt was encompassing the bigger picture. They were using empirical evidence used in previous outbreaks, compared to focusing on irregular marker responses such as containing the reproduction rate of Covid 19 at any cost. The "R" (rate of transmission) as it was known, is an incomplete measure of the true cost and benefit that is needed to be balanced with the impact on public health outcomes, of poverty, lack of access to healthcare, and basic services.

According to Swedish epidemiologist, by the middle of June, it was predicted there would be no more daily cases of the virus in Western Europe. However, in France and Spain two of the worst-hit counties, only 5% of the population had developed immunity, whereas in Stockholm it was estimated that 40% of the population was immune, as a result of letting the virus spread in the active (young and healthy) population.

The Guardian ran a daily berating of Sweden saying that it was irresponsible and their strategy was putting the economy before lives. The "lives versus economy" argument became a major talking point and lockdown fanatics would react angrily to even considering that the benefits of maintaining the economy and saving peoples livelihoods was as important.

Suddenly, having an opinion that attempted to balance risk and benefit which disagreed with the current status quo, was not acceptable, and anyone who argued, was caught in a straw man argument, that painted them as a right-wing, genocidal killer for even considering a fresh approach.

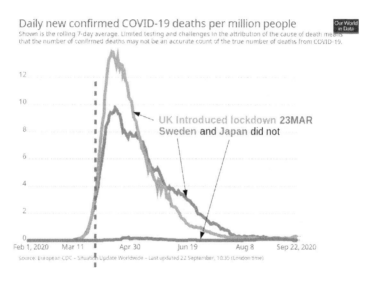

Graph comparing the UK that locked down, with Sweden and Japan who only made recommendations to citizens.

Whatever It Takes

Weighing up the cost of the lockdown is a legitimate question. Anyone who owns a business will tell you that if expenditure exceeds income over a long period, it is not sustainable. It has been reported that the daily cost of lockdown is £2.4 billion a day which is the cost of three new hospitals every day.

Analysts predict that the longer we are in lockdown, the less likely a V shape recovery will happen, which will scar the economy long term. The impending contraction of GDP could cause more wealth devastation and secondary deaths which far outweigh the lives saved by the lockdown. Could the cure be worse than the virus itself? Has anyone in government close to the decision making raised this issue?

The reality is that a deep recession could kill more people than the outbreak of the virus. In our attempt to 'protect the NHS', we are risking being unable to fund a future NHS in its current form. If the annual budget for the NHS (£133 billion/funded by GDP) is put at risk, this could drive down the standard of care available. Instead of saving the NHS or making the service better, our actions could make the service far worse than anyone has considered.

If the lockdown is a prolonged on /off strategy for 18 months (or a long term 'new normal' of how we view flu viruses) as suggested, the UK economy has been predicted to shrink by 25% (according to The Daily Telegraph) over the next two years. "I'm worried that in order to solve one problem we'd create a bigger problem," says Phillip Thomas a professor of risk management at Bristol University. In April 2020, the government borrowed more money than they did in the whole of 2019. The world's cash flow has dried up and there are bound to be serious consequences.

The government devised monetary incentives for businesses and employees so that they would accept the lockdown in a "whatever it takes" attitude. Grants, loans, and furlough schemes were implemented to save businesses and livelihoods. These incentives would have been useful if the economy could have returned to normal as soon as possible. However, the longer that it took, the more likely businesses on the edge would collapse and go under.

The furlough scheme alone was predicted to have reached over 9 million people. The workforce was given an incentive not to work. It was unsustainable for the state to pay the wages of millions of people indefinitely for jobs that may not exist anymore. The government used borrowed money to finance the furlough and other schemes, effectively robbing Peter to pay Paul. This money needs to be paid back with higher inflation, a devalued currency, or higher taxation. A vicious cycle could develop where businesses close, causing unemployment to rise and resulting in fewer people to pay taxes.

How many people were not working and supporting lockdown because the situation benefitted them? Seeing the wood through the trees is difficult when you are being paid 80% of your wages to stay at home? The government had created fairy tale policies that were only ever time limited. The reality was that many businesses faced not reopening because lockdown had choked them to death and many livelihoods will be lost. Figures from April 2020 showed one in 9 people were now out of work; unemployment was racing to record levels. Job vacancies were collapsing at their fastest rate; this left those being made unemployed nowhere to go apart from applying for universal credits.

Industries are collapsing, unable to cope with the restrictions not conducive to business. The jobs market is predicted to become sparse and highly competitive. The economic scarring could be so bad that we need to rethink how we view employment. Our life purpose in modern times had been entwined with our careers. In the future, as a consequence to the government's actions there may not be enough jobs for everyone, and having a livelihood may become a privilege, leaving the question how will people survive?

Only with the costs and benefits of different policy choices, can we make wise and effective long term decisions.

Protect the NHS

The conversation evolved from lives versus cost, into lives versus lives debate. By locking down society and encouraging people to stay at home there was an even bigger problem approaching. For every person that was dying of Covid 19, there was a negative inverse of excess deaths (estimated 20,000 in the first three months) from medical conditions such as heart disease and cancer because they were unable to access the care they needed.

Patients too fearful to visit hospital were dying when they would have likely lived if they had received the appropriate intervention. Over this period the A+E numbers dropped to a record low. The stay at home messaging was working too well and not in a good way. The UK had 50,000 more deaths than previous years during March and April, versus 27,000 reported Covid 19 deaths in the same period.

They moved tested/untested elderly patients from hospitals to care homes to clear bed spaces. These actions inadvertently caused an outbreak in 70% of care homes and made up 40-50% of all mortality for Covid 19 in the first three months.

We basically dumped a large sample of people back into care homes that were contagious with Covid 19, to avoid overwhelming the NHS. For the rest of us staying at home, lockdown was futile a) the peak number of cases had already happened by the start of lockdown on March 23rd b) in the government's attempts to avoid overwhelming the NHS they inadvertently overwhelmed the care homes instead. Up to 40-50% more people of Covid 19 mortality, would have survived had this not happened. Logically they cannot claim their actions saved lives.

Enter the race for a vaccine

The UK government had invested £300 million since the beginning of the outbreak to develop a Covid 19 vaccine. Bill Gates is coordinating seven vaccine factories across the globe, hedging his bets that a few would fail and one or two would succeed. The Jenner Institute in Oxford set up the first trial in April 2020 which promised to produce 100 million doses by the end of the year. Matt Hancock, the Health Secretary told the nation that a vaccine was the only option to save us from further restrictions.

However at the point of writing, we are a couple of weeks from rolling out these vaccines and instead of lifting restrictions, we are still locked down and are told that anyone one that doesn't accept the vaccine will be restricted further. They will not be able travel, attend concerts, sporting events or even work. Today labour has insisted to outlaw anyone with opposing views to vaccines.

In the quest for a vaccine, thousands of clinical trials were suspended, meaning patients will wait longer for new therapies. Just one-quarter of the National Institute for Health Research was going ahead as usual. Nearly six out of ten clinical trials are to be stopped entirely.

The vaccine was a hot topic and was touted by mainstream media as the only solution to ending restrictions. Some have expressed they will be first in the queue when the vaccine is ready but if so, please consider a) the vaccines are being rushed through testing faster than ever before b) the virus is rapidly mutating and has done so 30 times at the time of writing (according to a blog by Dr Sherri Tenpenny on her website Vaxxter). She wrote that a vaccine created in a trial today, will likely be all risk and no benefit by the time it reaches the market.

Vaccines are like a modern-day choice between heaven and hell. Early Christians were told that if they followed the rules and they were good on earth, they would enter heaven. However, if they broke the rules they would go to hell. It seems we are fallible to the idea of doing what is asked of us by our leaders because a reward is given at the end. Even if that reward doesn't exist, we are still compelled to comply.

History repeats itself

Although we have been led to believe this is a unique situation, pandemics and viruses are nothing new. This is just another novel flu virus of short duration, that when we are healthy, we are highly likely to recover with no long term effects. For instance, there were three large pandemics last century and Covid 19 is a flu virus extremely similar to those. The difference this time is our reaction to this virus in comparison to previous viruses.

Extended lockdowns are a new and untested strategy to manage pandemics. The only modern example in western history is the swine flu outbreak in Mexico in 2009 when school and businesses were closed which was abandoned after 18 days because of the mounting social and economic costs. Let's take a look at a couple of examples from the past;

Spanish Flu

The Spanish flu killed approximately 20-50 million people worldwide and 200,000 in the UK. Citizens were ordered to wear face masks but shops stayed open, contrary to many journalists today telling us there was a full lockdown. Opening times of stores were staggered to slow down possible transmission.

The virus appeared in the spring of 1918 and then returned in the fall that same year. It was first observed in Europe and unusually affected younger people, causing more US soldiers to die of the flu than in battle during World War I.

The public health advice in the 1918 pandemic was to sleep with your bedroom window open and spend time outside in fresh air and sunshine. Dr Richard Hobday author of "The Healing Sun: Sunlight and Health in the 21st Century" said, "Hospitals and patients who were nursed outside in tents and put in the sun seem to have recovered far better than those indoors."

Fever hospitals were still around from the time of smallpox and other outbreaks. Patients were kept there in separation from the uninfected patients. By the summer of 1919, the flu pandemic came to an end.

Asian flu 1957-58

You may not have heard of H2N2 as news outlets let this flu past as if nothing had happened, in contrast to Covid 19, which has dominated media outlets for the last six months.

The death toll worldwide was 1.5-4 million people which equates to 3-6 million people today, making Covid 19 look like the common cold. This flu was particularly lethal to 5-39 year olds which is the opposite to Covid 19. It was a ruthlessly quick process because 70% of victims were dead within 48 hours of reaching hospital.

Back then there was a stoic attitude to illness, perhaps because most people of the time had lived through the Second World War. If a person was sick they would isolate by going to bed, get better then return to work. The government devolved most of the operational day to day responsibilities of the pandemic to local authorities instead of centrally controlling from parliament.

Life went on as normal apart from changes that were regional and justified such as schools in London were closed at the height of the outbreak because this was where the highest concentration of cases were, based on hospital admissions and mortality rate. If something was cancelled it was because at a local level they had decided and not a central government making nationwide decisions based on regional data. This is a world away from daily briefings from the cabinet and indiscriminate national lockdowns.

Hong Kong Flu 1968-72

The H3N2 strain commonly known as Hong Kong flu spread around the world in the summer of 1968 and would return for the next three winters. By 1970, 1 million people had died worldwide and 80,000 in the UK. In a similar way to the current contagious Corona virus, when healthy people were infected the symptoms were mild and many recovered within a few days but symptoms were much worse in the elderly.

The Government's advice was much the same as today but without locking down society. People still went to work but were advised to wash their hands, maintain space between each other by avoiding public transport and walking where possible. It is estimated that the workforce lost a million man-hours in production but by refraining from shutting down the economy, the country was able to avoid a recession. It was a very British "stiff upper lip" approach of taking precautions but carrying on with life.

As more was known about the virus's transmission, dynamics, and aetiology, they realized that it wasn't as deadly as previously thought, much like Covid 19. There were fears there would be no immunity even after recovery but this virus proved to be like many others.

A vaccine became available but was in short supply and initially reserved for key workers. After the production of the vaccine was ramped up the severity of the virus was known and they weren't widely adopted, therefore spare vaccines were shipped abroad.

Go out and live your life.

The lockdown showed us how arbitrary and ridiculous some rules and regulations are, as well as the state's enforcement of them. Hopefully, you can now see that science is more fluid until the weight of data proves the theory. Even then we have to be careful because people with invested interest, people who stand to profit from proving the theory, can knowingly or unknowingly bias the science.

The most significant part of the reaction to the virus has been the disproportionate damage done by the cure (lockdown measures), relative to the harm caused by the virus. To fully understand what happened and why Covid 19 became the biggest global event since the 9/11, an independent investigation of the origins of the virus needs to be carried out and those at fault need to be held accountable.

Part II: Lockdown's efficacy

As time goes on it is becoming clearer that lockdown was a mistake when compared to its benefits. Through scientific bias, the virus was estimated to be deadlier than it actually was and we now know the death rate is closer to 0.1-0.26%. We also know that the vast majority of the population will be asymptomatic or will develop symptoms and recover. If you do not already have a chronic underlying condition, your chances of dying from Covid 19 are miniscule.

Locking down the population prolongs the problem because immunity is not build up in the community. Herd immunity is a proven science, where infected individuals produce whole cell/memory immunity. Not only do they become immune but they stop person to person spread in future waves. Letting younger people and low-risk groups become exposed to the virus helps to shield the vulnerable, by reducing the R figure. As opposed to a population with no memory immunity, the virus will continue to spread through all age groups.

Excess deaths occurred because all the focus was on suppressing the virus while other medical care could not be accessed. Non-essential care was abruptly stopped which prevented the diagnosis of life-threatening diseases. Cancer patients, for example, were unable to make follow up appointments, which created a huge backlog of patients waiting for vital treatment.

Professor Gupta from Oxford University says the lockdown has been highly ineffective, "In almost every context we've seen the epidemic grow, turn around and die away — almost like clockwork. Different countries had had different lockdown policies, and yet what we've observed is almost a uniform pattern of behaviour which is highly consistent with [our] model."

She also thought the long-term harm of protecting ourselves from exposure to pathogens in our day to day life made us more vulnerable to killer viruses, not less. Remaining in a state of lockdown was extremely dangerous for the vulnerability of the entire population to new pathogens. As the old wife's tale goes, 'dirt is good for us'.

Lastly, lockdowns are a luxury for middle classes on higher income who are more likely to be able to work from home and at the expense of lower-income workers, who are more likely to have jobs that need to be physically attended.

Falling below the standard expected of a government

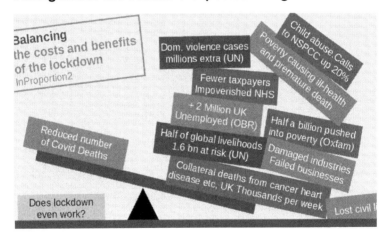

Taken from http://inproportion2.talkigy.com/

The list of the government's failings would be too long for this book, but I'll attempt to summarise them here:

Laws were created to force us to "stay home" and only leave our homes when absolutely necessary. This went against known facts that sunlight, social interaction, and quality of life are as significant to staying healthy and/or recovering from viruses. The government's advice caused panic and hysteria, which again left people susceptible to illness. People were forced to close their businesses, cancel plans, unable to visit loved ones from other households.

The second part of the slogan was to "protect the NHS". When did a public funded institution paid for through national insurance contributions become the nation's job to protect? The NHS is funded through our taxes so that if we ever need to access crisis and emergency care, this is available to us. We are guaranteed a flu season every winter by virtue of the climate of the UK, this means the NHS is used to a large influx of patients, the system has always been able to handle this in previous years. In my view it is the government's job to run the NHS effectively and not the general public's 'civic duty' to avoid accessing the NHS, as the current health sectary of state keeps telling us.

By paradox their decisions will put more pressure on the NHS in the long run than had they taken no action. "Protecting the NHS" has turned into record backlog of patient's on waiting lists for procedures because of missed appointments throughout lockdown. The third part was "save lives". During the lockdown people with life threatening symptoms were unable to access emergency care and died as a consequence. The UK had one of the largest excess deaths in Europe.

Large amounts of untested elderly people in hospitals were returned to care homes to make room for fresh Covid 19 cases, causing a mass outbreak of the virus to 'at risk groups' in care homes. This devastating act contributed to care homes accounting for more than 40-50% of virus's mortality rate in the first three months. Ask yourself this question if the government had taken no action, what percentage do you think would have died in care homes? By putting these people back into care homes meant these people died directly from Covid 19, that in my mind, would be still be alive otherwise.

Another estimated 20,000 people died as a result of not being able to access the healthcare system. By my math, 40,000 died in the first three months, up to 20,000 people died in care homes (hypothetically they would still be alive had we taken no action), another 20,000 would still be alive because they could access healthcare, by this logic we would have saved 40,000 lives had there been no action taken.

The government has been criticized for not locking down sooner and perhaps this is why they are still enforcing irrational and inconsistent restrictions. I believe this policy was wrong from the beginning. This sunk cost fallacy is from a false assumption that the virus was more deadly than in reality.

In my opinion we need to learn to live with the virus just like we do with many other viruses. We need to let the active population get back to work and let the vulnerable make their own choices as to what risks they are willing take, whilst taking all reasonable measures to support them.

When I read the story about the outbreaks in universities, instead of damning students, like most news outlets did, I felt that this was a blessing in disguise based on my assumption of what's known of other corona viruses. If students are spreading the virus amongst themselves they will develop whole cell/memory immunity which means, when they come into contact with Covid 19 in future they will be protected and also they will stop person to person spread therefore, protecting at risk groups.

The case for future lockdowns is weak. Professor Giesecke who helped craft an alternative approach in Sweden, has been a critic of further heavy restrictions by governments, saying that most people will eventually be infected. "A lockdown only pushes the severe cases into the future, it will not prevent them". The time to eradicate the virus has passed. It would appear the virus is here to stay.

He has also spoken about lockdowns being a privilege to richer nations. He said "you have to be careful with lockdowns in poor countries, as they create more problems than they solve". Lockdown in poor nations is more likely to result in life expectancy to fall and poverty to rise.

According to the Prof Udi Qimron at Tel Aviv University 99.9% of the world that has contracted Covid 19 has survived the virus which prompted him to say "in a world where decision makers, their advisers, and the media were unable to admit their mistake and the initial panic that gripped them, we would have long since returned to routine".

I am concerned that nobody in government is properly balancing the economic and social effects of the lockdown, in terms of the poverty and social unrest that could arise from total focus on suppressing a flu virus at all costs. When Matt Hancock was challenged regarding the possibility of 150,000 excess deaths caused by the lockdown he replied, "This didn't form part of the analysis." Is focusing on one or two metrics and excluding other data from the analysis, the best policy? This, in my opinion, is not following the science; it is cherry-picking the science and the refusal to look at the wider picture.

The government has set a precedent now that they are prepared to halt our lives at a moment's notice by decree of a few government ministers, who are openly only focused on one or two metrics, instead of taking a wider view i.e. not fully balancing the risks at hand.

What we really need is leadership that can stand by their decisions instead of changing their minds at every step.

Schools had been closed for six months, even though throughout July only 4 regions made up for 90% of Covid 19 deaths. This type of disproportionate nationwide intervention from central government is difficult to make sense of when compared to the risks.

When winter comes how is the UK government going to distinguish between one strain of flu and another? From what I understand from the testing there is a problem that the Covid 19 strain cannot be isolated from other flu strains. Will people with a seasonal cough be sent home until their test results return? Judging by the decisions made in spring and summer this could be a long winter of knee jerk reactions, without consulting a wider scope of specialists, lacking consideration to the consequences to people's livelihoods and ways of life.

If people are in an at-risk group then shield those individuals, but still allow them to make their own choices. As individuals, they are entitled to assess their own risks and decide for themselves how they wish to live their lives. It is not, in my opinion, the job of the state to order them to stay home and remove their freedoms. Give the recommendations, explain the risk and then let people make their own choice.

Elon Musk said it best with "If somebody wants to stay in their house, that's great and they should be able to, but to say they cannot leave their house and they will be arrested if they do, that's fascist. That is not democratic."

Imagine a government of yesteryears ever passing a law that declared you can only see certain members of your family at Christmas because of a flu virus? It would have been considered nothing more than absurd. Today it's a case of accepting this nonsense or breaking the law. We need a collective message that balances the risk with also appropriate action that our constitute members of parliament can debate. They also need to be able to vote on our behalf for new laws such as the rule of six.

This government has become what they said they wanted to remove from parliament. Before they were elected, they warned us about project fear and how they would remove the power from the few elite, to create an egalitarian society. Yet what we see seems to be a continuation – even deterioration – of the status quo.

Future restrictions

The government decided to lockdown for an intended three weeks so that the health services were not overwhelmed and to ensure sufficient capacity was available. However, 3 weeks was extended to 12 weeks and restrictions are on-going (8 months later), such as social distancing and the enforced wearing of masks, even though during the summer some regions of the UK had less than 10 cases per 100,000 people.

The evidence on masks is inconclusive to whether they will have an impact on stopping the spread of a virus or if in fact wearing them for prolonged period is damaging to our health. Surgical masks worn by a surgeon will change their masks every 20 minutes, how many people are changing their masks every 20 minutes? We do not yet understand the effects of wearing masks for prolonged periods without changing them. The full impacts of using masks in this way are unknown and could be doing more harm than good.

I would like to finish by saying that my deepest sympathies go out to anyone that has lost a loved one to the virus. In my analysis I've made judgment's that could be conceived callow, however they are meant with an authentic intentions that I felt balanced the risk between lives lost, protecting our freedoms and our culture, that our ancestors fought hard to preserve.

PART TWO

Patient A
Presenting symptoms: Apathy and malaise
Diagnosis: Commonsense paralysis caused by
pharmaceutical overload
Recommendation: teach them holistic principles
Prognosis: Full recovery expected

Chapter 4 – Movement is medicine

An active lifestyle is a simple answer to many of the major health challenges facing us today. If exercise was a pill, it would be considered a wonder drug because of all the benefits we get from being active. Imagine if being active was marketed in this way how many more people would be partaking in regular exercise? That would require a quantum leap in redesigning a proactive healthcare model.

Being active has the potential to reduce all-cause mortality and improve life expectancy. When we consider our reaction to Covid 19 and the emphasis placed on saving the NHS, wouldn't promoting exercise and setting up referral pathways for patients, be a much more logical way to ease the burden on the NHS?

The benefits of physical activity have been well documented. If a person carries out 30 minutes of moderate exercise such as walking at least five times a week, it can prevent and help manage over 20 chronic conditions including coronary heart disease, strokes, diabetes (type 2), cancer, obesity, mental health problems and musculoskeletal conditions.

Despite the multiple health gains connected to moderate exercise, half the population do not achieve the weekly amount suggested by the Chief Medical Officer to benefit from an active lifestyle. High levels of inactivity put a significant economic burden on the NHS due to treatment of long term health conditions that could be managed through exercise.

Instead of becoming more active as a population, we are becoming more inactive when compared to the 1980s. Back then we were 25% more likely to travel on foot or bike, today we watch twice as much TV, play less sport and are more sedentary. Through the convenience of technology, our lifestyles are becoming less physically demanding, resulting in us becoming less active.

The good news is that building up to just half an hour a day of moderate activity, several times a week can help to unlock a range of health benefits. This could be something as simple as walking instead of driving. After a few weeks, you could notice a significant difference in how you feel and also experience an increase in your energy levels.

Other benefits of a consistently active lifestyle are maintaining a healthy weight for a better shape and appearance and becoming stronger and fitter, which improves confidence and increases the opportunity for fun with family and friends.

Being active is defined as a movement which expends calories and raises our heart rate. When we are younger, we usually experience this when playing sport. There are three types of physical exercise; light, moderate and vigorous intensity. Moderate intensity is characterized by being able to talk but noticing that your breathing becomes quicker and deeper, your body warms up, your face has a healthy glow, and your heart beats faster than normal but without racing.

Intensity during activity will be different for everyone depending on their fitness levels. As a person increases their fitness levels they can achieve more because the activity becomes easier. Someone once gave me this advice when looking to improve their fitness; "it's not fun exercising when you're not fit, but when you're fit, exercise becomes fun."

Many people believe they just don't have the time to become more active. They feel too tired, too old or too unfit; these are just some examples of the reasons that stop people from being active. Another perception is that living an active lifestyle means training for the Olympics, which can often put people off before even getting started. However, a non-competitive active lifestyle is a lot easier than you think. Becoming fit is about identifying where you are right now and then setting appropriate and realistic goals for you, which we will explore in this chapter.

Let's Get Moving

Before I became a Chiropractor I had a successful personal training business. I was gifted the opportunity to work with the NHS on a pilot scheme for exercise referral called, "Let's Get Moving." This has since been rolled out nationally with UK Active. My role was to work closely with GP's and their patients as a bridge to helping them become more active.

It was the first scheme of its kind. The idea was to place exercise at the heart of the NHS as a core business rather than a peripheral concern. This was characterised as a holistic behavioural change programme of physical activity, which provided a systematic approach in supporting adults to become more active, for the prevention and management of chronic disease related to inactivity.

The pathway was designed for GP's to select patients that were not meeting the recommendations for an active lifestyle. They would then make an appointment with me to explore realistic goals for them. A typical session included figuring out their starting point, understanding and working on overcoming barriers to exercise, developing an activity plan and dealing with possible relapses.

The patients that were referred were very different to my personal training clients. They mostly had underlying health conditions such as obesity, diabetes, and heart disease or addiction issues. Many were in no position to join a gym because of their poor health, which limited the range of exercise that was safe and available to them. In many cases they were completely inactive before the first session.

It was clear from the beginning that this project was about getting them onto the first rung of exercise, and not in the short term to participate in a Triathlon. The goal of the initial meeting was to assess what they could do without risking their health further. Then figure out the type of person they were to motivate them effectively.

The coaching was not about what was said but more about how it was said. We were taught to use motivational interviewing. This is where the coach and participant are equal to one another. The coach uses questions to draw the answers from the participant through self-awareness. By answering questions participants were able to gain insight for themselves.

So instead of stating that exercise is good for us because of x, y and z, the coach would ask "Why is exercise good for us?" By working in this way, we could discover the level of knowledge of the participant and this would also tell us more about their psychology. The participant would then be encouraged to reflect on their situation and belief structures without judgment or criticism.

When the answer comes from the participant, they were more likely to follow through positively and take responsibility for their goals. As their coach, I was acting as their internal dialogue, challenging their current belief structures. For example, I might ask, "When was the last time you were active?" The patient may respond by answering when they were younger. Then I might explore why they stopped exercising and they might say "I just don't have time anymore."

Is time the issue? Or is it just a surface level excuse? Perhaps they do not value exercise as a priority and therefore do not make time to exercise? Whatever we value most is how we choose to spend our time. To change the value system there has to be a shift in a person's belief structures that created the barrier. Through identifying the subconscious barriers to exercise which usually only appear underneath the surface level, only then can real change and transformation be made. This can only happen if the person feels comfortable opening their inner feeling to the coach, which is why the language and integrity of the coach is vital in this approach.

Once I'd discovered a barrier, the next step is to understand why they are there. It isn't always for the reasons we presume. Some people might find that underneath a barrier like "not having enough time", the real reason they didn't exercise was that they felt depressed or self-conscious.

Helping the participant to deconstruct their barriers was always a powerful experience for participant. When someone gained insight into themselves by discovering a key to unlock a negative pattern or behaviour, there was energy in the room that felt like something special was happening. When people talked openly, freely and truthfully I always felt lightness and a feeling of heightened consciousness.

By helping people to understand the meaning behind their current belief structures that shape their lives, it can open up the space to let go of old beliefs that do not serve them and allow new beliefs to form. If they can reach these conclusions themselves, they are more likely to follow through on them than if they are just told them by an authority figure.

The common assumption is that if a patient is given instructions or made to feel concerned, or even fearful for their health, this is the best way to get results with them. Practitioner's own beliefs and aspirations for a patient often determine how we interact with them. By seeking to "fix" the patient, motivated by a desire to help, but in doing so could undermine self-directed behavioural change. As long as practitioners have these beliefs towards changing people's behaviour, they will continue to have limited results.

Judging ourselves and our environment is part of life. We are constantly making conscious and unconscious judgments every day. In the traditional practitioner/patient setting, the practitioner makes judgments and a decision based on what they think is best for the patient. The patient's motives, however, are more likely to trigger successful change than any general advice practitioners could give. Therefore, it would be best to take an interest in the patient's concerns and values without judgment before giving their advice.

In this way, the advice is considered to be individualised and more far-reaching. The patient is more likely to act on the advice given if it is relevant and achievable to them.

Practitioners would be there to help them realise what stops them from moving forward and taking positive action in their lives. They need to decipher what is controlling or determining their decisions and the practitioner needs to support them by shining a light on their emotional blocks so that they can overcome them.

If you use a forceful attitude to try and change someone, don't be surprised if they respond with resistance. However, if the conversation is conducted in such a way that the guidance was their idea, they are more likely to comply. When people feel understood they are less likely to resist. To help them change you have to meet them where they are at.

We have all wronged people when we think we are right or believe we have a superior point of view. The tendency is to jump in when we disagree with what is being said, is very tempting. The desire to correct a discrepancy between how things are and how we think they ought to be is a natural part of being human. When we make others feel wrong, they are more likely to become defensive. However, when we gently guide them to arrive at their conclusion, they feel more confident and empowered.

How many people do you know who strongly resist when they are told they must do something? When resistance happens, the advice is often ignored or followed with resentment because the person feels as though their sense of control is being taken away. They will often argue defiantly, interrupt and negate to try and avoid that loss of control.

When this happens they will become defensive and they will care less about what you think regardless if you feel you're acting in their best interests. The person in this scenario would more likely become entrenched and belligerent in their position to avoid change than embracing change. This is the surface level belief structure protecting the more vulnerable, deeper held beliefs about themselves. Approaching a person in this way lacks rapport and trust to pass the surface level, which is needed for long term, self-directed, behavioural change.

In my opinion the solution is to change the role of the practitioner to be a part physician and part psychologist. By learning to recognise the patient's ambivalence is not because of a lack of insight, knowledge or concern but rather their lack of change is because of their unresolved ambivalence.

This was confirmed to me by a friend who was a doctor. He had studied for six years and eventually became a GP but as he progressed within the medical profession, he developed a more holistic approach. He realized that improving emotional health by working on self-esteem, as well as diet and exercise, is more important than the recommendations of conventional medicine.

Once he realized he was conflicted by working in a system that he wasn't aligned with, he decided to leave the profession and began a coaching business. He still wanted to work with people but in a way that felt more congruent to him. I have heard stories like this many times, where student doctors with a genuine willingness to help people, drop out of the profession because the realise the limitation of the current healthcare system.

The practitioners of the future will use a guiding style, listening for "change" talk. When patients use self-motivating phrases that can be natural markers of readiness to change, practitioners would then act on this. The patient may express willingness by saying "I would like to," or "I could do that". They may have reasons formulated or realise a need or importance specific to them. The practitioner's role would be to help fast track the patient into self-determined commitments.

In NLP they call this "lead and follow." This means that in the beginning, the conversation is led by the practitioner but then switches to the patient leading and the practitioner follows. The patient, not the practitioner expresses the concern about their behaviour and formulates their arguments in favour of change. This allows the patient to step into their power because they take responsibly of being the decision-maker, guided by the practitioner.

One of the first questions to ask yourself is, "How important is it that you become more active?" Then score that with a number from 1-10. If you were working with me, I might ask, "Why not a higher number?" or "What would need to happen for it to become more important for you to be active?"

Your answers will reveal what type of person you are and the best way to motivate you. Some people might say it is because of their health or because they want to be a better parent. These distinctions are important as they say a lot about the person's innate motivations, which guide the conversation to target the best results for them.

Depending on the situation they might say they would like to drink less alcohol or stop binge eating. I would always search deeper to find out the root cause of the issue. This could then be stated in a positive way to anchor to during challenging times. When a person says they want to stop something they are addicted to, they will always revert to the addiction if they do not overcome the driver/cause of the behaviour. The addiction is a coping mechanisms used to deal with stress, so if you can find out the deeper cause and address that, achieving the smaller goals will become easier.

The root cause of the problem won't be the first response you receive, as the answer is always beneath the surface. If a practitioner has asked questions in a non-judgmental way, creating a safe space for them to open themselves to the underlying issue that they may not even be aware of, will help them to become self-aware. The environment needs to feel safe for them to open up and allow their vulnerability to appear, instead of clinging in defensiveness to their coping mechanisms. From this place, they are more likely to change or address the deeper reasons for their behaviour, it sometimes surprised me what they revealed.

Once the motivation for someone is established, it's time to discover what is stopping them from achieving what is important to them. I might ask, "What would make you more confident if you did decide to change?" They might respond, "If I had a clear plan." In this phase, we are attempting to deal with the objection in a positive way. By continuing with this brainstorming we are testing the practicality of how they can realistically maintain their behavioural change.

Once I'd found what motivates a person, visualisations were a powerful tool that could be tailored to the individual. For example, if a person wants to become more active so they can play with their children more often, a positive future would be for them to imagine playing with their children, listening to sounds, how they would feel and what they would see. It is important to feel like they are already there. Then we would switch to a future where they do not act or no change occurs. It's important that they feel the pleasure of change but it is equally important that they experience the pain of not acting.

We all have subprograms that help us make decisions. For example, most people will want to move away from pain to gain pleasure. For them to change they need to have the pain attached to a visualization of a possible future where they can see what will happen if they don't act. Others need more positive reinforcement by focusing on a positive future of what can happen if they do change. I found the former was more likely to apply to patients with addictive tendencies.

When we sit down or think about a task we normally start with the goal in mind. However, when going through this process of figuring out what is important to us first, the goal becomes more specific, realistic and individual to us. This is the point when we would start to set goals. Once the person indicates and feels ready to start an exercise program and is clear why they are committing themselves to doing so, we would help them put together a 12 week activity program.

We would then summarize the plan by recapping their reasons and integrating those reasons into their lives. We would also discuss things that could get in the way and how they would overcome them if they materialized. This might include setting boundaries with themselves or others. This would lead on to how other people could help to support them and finishing with when and how they would know they've achieved success.

People have to be met at the place they are currently at. Change for some people could just be getting out and walking each day, or for others, it could be acknowledging that they aren't yet ready for change but leaving them with the seed to change when they are ready. One of the best insights I had working on this project was to scale back what I wanted from the meeting and instead focus on what the patient was prepared to change. Hopefully it's clearer now that the reason we or someone we know is unmotivated to be active is not because of laziness or a lack of time, it's because of our or their unresolved ambivalence.

Preparing For Exercise

As we become older, we generally move less and this can result in stiff joints and muscles. A lot of people put this down to old age, which is a natural process that happens to all of us. When we are young and healthy our joints usually have the correct range of movement but when we age or move less, the range of our joints can reduce. This is why we experience stiffness and/or more susceptible to injury.

Replacing the shape of your posture with natural symmetry of square shoulders, level hips, head central and from the side standing upright without twisting, is the best place to start before conducting any exercise program. One of the busiest times to see new patients at our chiropractic clinic is in February. This is because many people start a gym program in January and by

February they either are experiencing a niggling injury or they have to stop exercising because of an injury.

When preparing your body for exercise it's important to understand the alignment of your posture to avoid unnecessary injury. The closer you are aligned to the correct geometric positions the stronger your foundation will be. However the more misaligned you are, the more likely you are to experience pain and injury. Our posture is a window to our spine. I sometimes say to patients, when they go home to stand in front of a mirror and spend a few moments just observing their posture. This is a really good way to begin to understand posture and spot where issues are.

Let's imagine when you look in the mirror, your shoulders are not level and one is more forward than the other (asymmetry). You then begin a generic gym program of symmetrical based exercises that may include bench press, an exercise which requires symmetry, equal strength on both sides of the body, it is more than likely that when you lift and lower the weight you will be reinforcing the imbalances that are already there, therefore making you more prone to injury.

This is why the shape of your posture is a factor, that will determine your entry-level point of activity. The closer you are to the midlines (upright and symmetrical), the more likely vigorous activity will be safe for you, but the further you are away from them the less appropriate they will be. When my patients ask my advice on what exercise they can do to help themselves, I normally say they can do whatever they like as long as it doesn't aggravate in any way. If it does then they must stop.

On the one hand, there is healing and on the other there are triggers. If you repeat too many triggers this will counteract how quickly the body heals and can eventually lead to injury or worsening an injury. The reason they must stop is that when they are repeating a trigger to a problem they are causing further micro trauma that cannot be healed faster than the injury is occurring. When someone is healing from an injury they need rest. If they just continue to repeat the trigger, it will further reinforce the imbalance of the body and will likely create poor movement patterns, which eventually make us even more susceptible to injury in the future.

Within your body, the nervous system acts like a collection of warning lights (pain sensors) that are only used when a problem such as a trigger or an injury arises. The pain is there to highlight the problem and immobilize the area so that further injury (muscle spasms) does not occur. Your body's autonomic patterning will sacrifice movement to protect the CNS encased within the spine and the structures that surround them.

When we feel pain or restricted movement, we can experience multiple compensation mechanisms such as tight hamstrings, lower back issues and rounded shoulders. These muscular compensations arise because of restrictions in the facet joints (the interlocking joint between the bones of the spine) and/or the loss of ability to shock absorb through the disc and spine. These compensations are like switching on the protection mode for your muscles. They help to restrict movement but if the movement is forced, pain will arise.

Over time compensations can affect our balance and coordination. Our brain's awareness of our joints does not match with our bodies built in patterns of movements which can cause further compensations. These are like bodily blind spots for our brains. When someone says they have poor balance or coordination and are otherwise healthy, the likelihood is that they will have compensatory movements due to restrictions between the facet joints.

Exercising our muscles can cause pain, which is normal. Our bodies may experience pain as a result of being challenged by exercise. There is another type of pain we may experience during exercise, when something doesn't feel quite right or when we have a nagging pain in our joints. Knowing the difference is important so that we can exercise safely. The body will only allow so much of the second type of pain before an injury occurs.

Take the scenario where someone is in the gym and they feel the second type of pain caused by a specific exercise. Most people will usually stop that exercise but in a small amount of cases they will continue because of their of lack awareness to this types of pain, which will in all likelihood make the injury worse. Knowing the difference between these pains is important to avoid unnecessary injury.

This is why correcting poor movement patterns is so important when undertaking an exercise program. If a person has been inactive for some time and has blind spots, hiding compensatory movements due to restricted joints, poor balance and coordination, the likelihood of injury is increased, therefore maintaining exercise as a long term solution will be difficult and could even make their situation worse.

Seeking advice from a professional such as a Chiropractor, Osteopath or Physiotherapist when starting an exercise program regardless of if a person is in pain or not, could help you understand your entry-level point to exercise and possibly prevent an injury. Some people will be able to jump straight into exercise and clear these compensations through movement alone but others will not.

Compensations can be corrected but they have to be done in a specific sequence in the same way that knots are untied. If you just randomly started untying a sequence of knots you could create more knots and this is what happens when we don't deal with the original compensation, we develop new ones. This is how people create poor movement patterns that cannot be solved through exercise alone.

In the untying knots analogy, the first knot to be untied is chosen to be the one which will allow the others to be unlocked in the quickest sequence. In holistic medicine, we call this the cause of the problem. Once this has been identified, the other compensations will be released by a similar sequence. The severity of the compensations will determine the length of the sequence needed to successfully free those areas.

Another option is to consider a personal trainer because they are taught to assess your current fitness levels and identify any abnormal movement patterns. They will design a fitness plan so that you can exercise safely and within your limits. With their guidance, you will be given specific exercises to counteract imbalances which progressively developed over time to achieve better posture.

Exercise is beneficial for everyone but not all exercise is good for everyone. The entry point for someone overweight with underlying health conditions is going to be different from a footballer returning from preseason. For the former, repeating the same high impact movements, again and again, like football training will increase the likelihood of injury or risking their health further, causing the person to be inactive for longer.

It would be better for them to begin walking several times a week and to build from there. This way they can build their cardiovascular fitness with minimal risk to injury. When walking, the range of movement needed is less important because the forces through the joints are of low impact. Over time, the range of movement would improve and allow the person to consider some more challenging types of activity.

One exercise that is highly beneficial for replacing a lost range of motion in joints is Yoga or Pilates. Yoga and Pilates of any kind is good for us and can be modified to suit all levels of fitness.

What to do next

Once you know your entry-level point as an individual, it is time to start a plan of action. The best way to achieve anything in life is to set clear goals. By doing this we are visualizing what we want to achieve in a set period.

When I worked in the fitness industry we used the acronym S.M.A.R.T which stands for Specific, Measurable, Achievable, Realistic and Time. This acronym can work for any activity. For example, if walking (specific and realistic) was your entry level you may decide to walk three times a week for 30 minutes (measurable and achievable) for the next month (time) before reviewing your progress. At this point, you could continue your current level of activity or decide to increase the frequency, duration and intensity because your fitness improved.

By achieving this level of fitness, this will help you gain the health benefits of living an active lifestyle. However, the level of intensity will have its limitations. If you are overweight and your goal is weight loss, the likelihood is this particular programme will not create the metabolic after burn which is essential for any weight loss programme.

Therefore fitness is a progression. If losing weight is your goal and your entry-level is walking, then once you become fitter and you are used to exercising again, the level can be increased. Your body is designed to move, the more you move over time, you will start to feel enjoyment from exercising.

Finding a partner or a group with similar fitness levels is a great way to stay motivated and make friends. They can also hold you accountable to your goals. If you are all in it together and you're sticking to your goals, an extra enjoyment will be felt with team mates. This can also strengthen commitment because you'll want to support the group by following through.

When I was in the recruit training for the Marines we would sometimes do physical training sessions 3-4 times a day. I was always interested in sport at school which is one of the reasons why I joined. When I was 17 years old I entered the careers office and they gave me an exercise program to follow which consisted of upper body workouts and running in military boots. This programme was designed to get me to the level of fitness needed to start recruit training.

The reason they give a predesigned workout programme is because to start recruit training you needed to be at a certain level of fitness from the beginning, which would progress to throughout training. At the end of 30 weeks recruits had to complete the commando tests which included the 6 mile endurance course, a 9-mile speed march, the Tarzan assault course and the 30 miler.

In the Marines we were always contending with each other to come first, especially when it came to fitness but what was more important was the group as a whole. If someone didn't achieve the correct standards, on most occasions the training team wouldn't just punish the individual, they would punish the whole group. I learnt very quickly that my behaviour has a consequence and affects not only me, but everyone around me.

Becoming fit is a journey and you can go as far or little as you are willing to go. Discovering what motivates you will be the strongest driving force on that journey. My motivation was I loved the challenge of taking on a project that pushed me both mentally and physically. As a young man, I wanted to see how far I could go. I look back fondly on those times because of the camaraderie in adversity and the realization that although it was painful at times, what I remember is the feeling of achievement with my peers.

There is lifelong confidence I take from this period of my life that permeates to every challenge I encounter. Becoming fit is not just about losing weight or getting more toned. It is about improving not only our health but also our self-esteem so that we can self-actualize who we are. Losing weight and improving your appearance is just a by-product of that process.

When we push ourselves consistently in a way which is ecological to our body's capability to a challenge, we are capable of achieving far more than we realise. Over time we start to feel better about ourselves and this imbues confidence within us. How far you want to go with it is up to you. If walking regularly is enough for you, know that you will still benefit long term.

Discover how to be your own coach by going through this questionnaire, to figure out your barriers, which will lead to your solution. To achieve the best results you need to reflect and control the decisions. These questions will discover the best way to motivate you and help you understand yourself better.

If you're coaching others through this questionnaire to make changes, draw the solution out, rather than giving them your advice too soon. This will allow them to buy into a partnership while maintaining their autonomy.

This is the questionnaire we used on the "Let's Get Moving" project;

Questionnaire

Importance

Look at the questions below and list the thing that comes to mind:

- How important is it for you out of ten to become more active?
- Why did you pick this number and not a lower number?
- What would need to happen for it to become even more important to you to become more active?
- If you have decided to change, how confident are you that you will manage to become more active and stay that way?
- Why did you pick this number and not a lower number?
- What might help you be more confident about living a more active lifestyle?
- What are the three most important benefits you would hope to see if you become more active?

Visualizations

- Spend a couple of minutes imagining a future where you decided to become more active and maintained an active lifestyle for the next 1-3 years. What would it be like for you? How might things be different?
- Spend a couple of minutes imagining a future where you decided to NOT become more active, stay the same or do less activity than you do now for the next 1-3 years. What would it be like for you? How might things be different?

List of activities

Walking

Bowls

Swimming

Playing sport, e.g. Badminton or football

Cycling

Going to the gym

Nature conservation

Gardening

Dancing

Yoga or Pilates

Name two or three activities from the list or a different activity not listed that you could start immediately.

Goal setting

If you did decide to become more active, what would you like to achieve or how would you like to be different in 3-4 months?

I will...
(insert activity)

On...(date)

At.........................(time)

At...(where)

For…………………………………………………………………………………….

(duration)…………………………………….(frequency/times a week)

Summary

- The reasons I want to be more successful are:
- I will know I have been successful when:
- This is what I am going to do to be successful:
- Other people can help me by:
- Things that might get in the way of my plan are:
- I will get round these by:

What if I am finding it difficult?

Now you have your goals and know why they are important to you. Some people will find becoming more active harder than others. Here are some suggestions which other people have found helpful in their efforts to become more active:

- Remind yourself of the reason you would like to become more active

- Keep these reasons (or your goals) somewhere you can see them

- Use a diary to record what you have done and how you improve

- Share your plans with others

- Become more active with other people, such as family or a friend

- Make sure activities are fun and enjoyable

- Join a group or a club

- Not being disheartened if you miss a session, remember to just keep going

- Book a consultation with a fitness professional

Further suggestions

Walking groups; a led walk with a trained walk leader, where you can meet new people and walk an interesting route, for all levels of ability. Check out Walking The Way To Health (whi.org.uk) or the Ramblers (ramblers.org.uk). This website might help you get started: (walkengland.org.uk/walknowgettingstarted.aspx)

Green exercise: including gardening, nature conservation and anything which involves getting active outdoors that helps improve your local environment. You could apply for an allotment through your local council or find out about conservation schemes through BTCV (btcv.org.uk).

Sports Club: local voluntary sports clubs where you can join in and meet others interested in your activity. Activities vary from football to kayaking to running to archery. Some sports offer introduction offers such as boot camps or Get Back into Netball.

Active travel: walking and cycling to work or the shops, or even a bit of the way. Try leaving your car at home or getting off the bus a stop early. This website helps you find walks in many cities (walkit.com).

Leisure centres: local authorities and private gyms where you can try out classes or just use the facilities to swim, practice yoga, dance or play tennis. You find out more on your local authority website or through the fitness industry association (fia.org.uk/choose-a-gym.html).

Parks and open spaces: lots of parks have facilities for ball games like basketball and tennis, as well as green space for walking, jogging, football and other activities. Check out couch to 5km (website insert here).

Cycling: whether that be on the roads or in the countryside, cycling is suitable for most fitness levels. For information on cycling routes go to sustrans.com or if you are feeling sociable britishcycling.org.uk for information on mass participant events.

Getting active safely: If you have underlying health conditions you may research further before embarking. Nhs.uk/livewell/fitness will give you more information on becoming more active or bhf.org.uk/keeping_your_heart_healthy/staying_active.aspx.

Chapter 5 – Eat your medicine

In the previous chapter, we talked about how exercise is extremely important in helping us live a healthier lifestyle. However, exercise is only one of the three pillars in lifestyle modifications, the second is diet. We need sufficient energy to survive and the fuel we choose determines our health as much as exercise, if not more. For every piece of muscle, bone or any other matter in our bodies to be formed, it has to be ingested first as a food source. Our digestive systems, convert this energy sources into living tissue so that we can grow and function. Therefore the food we eat dictates our health.

Have you ever heard people say, "We are what we eat?" The impact of what we eat and how it affects our health cannot be ignored. Understanding the science of food is essential to achieving optimum health. I believe that most medical symptoms caught in the early stages can be managed through diet and supplementation. This can avoid long term medication that more often than not relieves symptoms but does not address the cause. Your diet is your life long medication.

Figures estimate that up to 50% of the population today suffer from a chronic disease. We are seeing an increase in cancer and obesity and the UK is one of the most medicated societies in the world. We consume more junk food and sugary foods than the rest of Europe. Worldwide more than 1 billion people are estimated to be overweight including 300 million that are obese.

As we age our diets become even more important because as our bodies begin to slow down, so does our metabolism. To illustrate the point, if a 30-year old sportsman successfully maintained his weight through diet and exercise, at 40 years old he would put on an extra 3.5kg a year if he still ate and exercised the same. This is what is commonly known as "middle-age spread". On top of that from our thirties onwards, we lose approximately up to 5% of muscle every year. Therefore, when we talk about a long term healthy lifestyle we must also include diet.

Despite education by governments, these trends are continuing to rise. Obesity is an early indicator of more serious conditions such as cancer, diabetes and respiratory disease. The NHS spends around 6 billion annually on health conditions related to weight problems and in 2019 there was 900,000 obesity, connected hospital admissions. The latest pandemic has highlighted that obese people are four times more likely to be hospitalized with Covid 19 than those without underlying health conditions.

The highest rates of obesity are associated with the lowest income areas in the UK. This is more than likely because they have a high concentration of fast food outlets and are limited for choice with outlets for fresh fruit and vegetables. Children in poverty by the age of 11 are three times as likely to be obese than their more privileged peers.

One in ten children starting primary school and one in five starting secondary schools are obese. We find ourselves spending millions of pounds putting people on the most cutting edge medication to manage this modern-day crisis but the problem isn't getting any better. The numbers are continuing to climb year on year.

What if this was preventable? What if the answer was a much simpler solution than drugs or surgery? Perhaps many diseases considered incurable by scientists and the medical profession could be managed or cured by what we eat? Does that sound farfetched to you? Eating a balanced diet of fresh fruit and vegetables and cutting out sugar and junk food has the potential to dramatically improve a person's poor health.

Let's do some myth-busting:

Myth number 1: People need more than vegetables to survive.

Truth: A balanced diet can be obtained by eating fresh fruit, vegetables, seeds and nuts. You will be much healthier if you keep to these food groups instead of eating processed and refined foods with many added ingredients.

Myth Number 2: Eating healthily is expensive.

Truth: Next time you go to the supermarket you can see for yourself that the cost of fresh fruit and vegetables is very reasonable and will cost a lot less than a diet of ready meals and takeaways.

Myth Number 3: It is too difficult to cook healthily.

Truth: It is easy to cook healthily if you keep it simple. Chopping ingredients up and stir-frying, roasting or steaming them is quick and nutritious. It is just having the confidence and motivation to do so.

Overfed and unnourished

Problems quite often begin when a person gets into bad habits of eating foods that are addictive. This means that they will overcome the internal signals that their stomach is full and will continue to eat and crave the food again, afterwards. Over time they will become overweight and because they are not eating live food sources, that grow with sunlight. When a person consumes foods that are devoid of nutrients, instead of live food sources that are full of nutrients, they will also become undernourished.

They will not be receiving what they need from their diet; therefore they are more prone to becoming sick and putting on weight. They have less energy and more prone to injury. They are less confident because of their appearance; therefore they go out less, so they receive less fresh air, sunlight, which makes them more prone to feeling depressed. In this example their health is on a decline long before they eventually develop symptoms that lead them to visit a doctor.

The cells

A fertilized egg is 96% water, a baby at birth is 80% water and a fully grown adult is 70% water. Our 70-100 trillion cells live in water universes inside us. They are individual oceans that adjoin and communicate with each other. Once upon a time, we lived in the ocean before moving to exist on landing grounds. Our cells are the living seas of the earth in human form.

The cells are just like us and need fuel to survive. What we eat and drink creates their environment. Healthy cells prefer natural products and this can show in our appearance. When someone looks healthy they will have good skin, healthy eyes and vibrant energy. However, when someone eats a lot of refined sugars and processed food, the cells become bogged down and unhealthy, which again shows in our appearance resulting in skin problems, dry hair and a lack of vibrancy.

This is another version of growth versus protection. When we eat toxic foods our cells will close the membrane doors to avoid harmful substances from entering. Over time our cells become overwhelmed as they sacrifice what they need to keep harmful substances from entering. When the cell becomes fatigued so does our appearance.

In contrast, when we eat foods that are beneficial to the cell, they open their doors and let them in. The cells receive what they need and have more energy to keep them in good working order which shows in our outward appearance. Our cells affect how healthy we are and they are affected by what we feed and the water they live in.

Most chronic diseases are caused by two major problems, toxicity and deficiency. The majority of processed junk food is highly toxic and devoid of nutrients. Over time when the environment that surrounds the cells are toxic and not receiving the fuel, vitamins and minerals they need, chronic symptoms will begin to occur.

The solution to healing a chronic illness is to first detoxify the body by making the cell environment less toxic and more alkaline. By understanding the difference between alkaline and acidic foods groups we can then make this a longer term solution to our diets. Secondly, we must start routinely testing our vitamin and mineral levels so that we know if our bodies are deficient of them and if they are, we replace them. Once you understand the cause, the solution is simple.

Healthy food groups

As a personal trainer, I was used to giving my clients a tailored diet plan by assessing the changes needed for their specific goals. However, when I worked with "Let's Get Moving" there was no dietary assessment time and it was virtually impossible to give accurate dietary suggestions to individuals. Many of my patients saw increasing their exercise and making changes to their diet as similar goals and therefore they would often ask me for dietary advice.

Instead of giving diet plans, I decided to draw up a generic list of food groups to either add to their diet or avoid. The list was split by alkaline versus acidic food groups. For example, processed sugar was on the 'avoid' (acidic) list and vegetables were on the 'add' (alkaline) list. I found this very beneficial and was pleased when I began to see people starting to think for themselves. It was also another way to move away from the harmful effects of calorie counting and focus more on the effects different food groups have on the body.

List of foods with healthy alternatives

Avoid	Add
Potatoes	Sweet potato/root vegetables
Pasta	Spelt/lentils/chickpeas
Rice	Brown/wild rice or quinoa
Bread	Spelt/rye sourdough bread
Hydrogenated oils	Coconut/rapeseed/olive/hemp oil
Margarine	Organic butter/goats butter
Table salt	Himalayan/sea salt
Daily fruit	Local seasonal fruit in moderation/not daily
Full fat milk	Semi-skimmed/coconut /almond/live yoghurt

BMI

Our weight is made up by the skeleton (bone density), organs, muscle, fat and water content. These components of our weight are all affected by our diet. If we eat more foods than our lifestyle demands, we will store that energy in our fat cells causing us to gain weight.

When the medical profession talks about people being overweight they are using Body Mass Index as a measurement, which calculates body composition. The Body Mass Index divides a person's height by their weight to determine if they are a healthy weight by working out their percentage of fat content.

The fat content of a healthy person is 18-25%. 25-30% is overweight and anything above 30% is considered obese. Athletes, for example, have the lowest fat content at 8-12% of body weight. However, if the fat content is below 5%, the immune system can be compromised making them prone to illness and infections. Fat in moderation is an important food type which is essential for good health.

There is a problem with the BMI in that is does not distinguish between fat, muscle and bone density. If someone had a higher muscle (which weighs more than fat) to fat content they could be considered overweight. For example, using this method the BMI of a bodybuilder with high muscle content would be considered overweight. Therefore for anyone with a high muscle content would need to interpret the BMI measurement with caution.

If you are overweight your body is put under more stress than someone with an ideal weight. The' engine room' of your body contains your organs and they have to work harder. Your joints are also placed under unnatural pressure which could lead to early wear and tear.

Food Groups

Although I think the BMI is a good tool to help understand your height to weight ratio, I tend not to focus on either the BMI or calorie counting. I believe that paying attention to particular food groups is more important. I find that when I receive a balanced diet and avoid unnatural foods I seldomly overeat, therefore putting on weight is not an issue.

Humans need six key nutrients for a wholesome and balanced diet. These are macronutrients (carbohydrates, proteins and fats) and micro-nutrients (vitamins, minerals and water). Macronutrients provide the fuel we need to grow and function, whereas micro-nutrients support our immune systems and ensure our cells are healthy. Both are crucial to our health and well-being.

Proteins are the building blocks of life. Amino acids are long strings of proteins made from DNA. The cell is made of proteins which are like little machines that help the cell carry out its functions.

When people think of addictions they normally think of alcohol or drugs. However addictions can be found in the foods we eat such as sugar, salt and fat. In nature, it is very rare for these three to be together in one food source but this is how most processed foods are made. The more they are mixed the more addictive they become. This is why people start to overeat when they are no longer satisfied with being full. Instead, they are chasing the chemicals and the feelings they gain from them. As a general rule, if you pick up a packet of food and don't recognize what is on the ingredient list then it is highly likely it's processed.

Like any addictive drug, it is never enough and the reason for this is because foods which are full of artificial sweeteners, preservatives and additives do not nourish us in the same way as natural food groups. When we eat a balanced diet we overeat less and we maintain our weight because our body is not being tricked by chemicals which are designed to confuse our taste buds.

Glucose

Glucose is blood sugar that has been broken down in the body. It is produced by natural sugars such as fruit, carbohydrates and refined sugars. Glucose is important for the body because it is a fast-acting energy source and useful in flight or fight responses or endurance exercise. Have you ever heard of anyone suggesting to someone who was running a marathon, to eat a bowl of pasta the night before? This is because pasta is a carbohydrate that can be stored by the body to produce fast-acting energy using glucose when our bodies become tired.

For this reason when we are exercising regularly carbohydrates in our diet can be burnt off as glucose. However, if we are consuming carbohydrates without working them off, we will ultimately gain weight as the glucose is kept in our fat stores. Insulin acts like a broom, sweeping up excess sugar from the bloodstream and depositing them in our liver or fat stores.

When a person's body has constant high blood sugar levels, it can cause the body over time, to become insulin resistant. This means that when their body releases insulin (the hormone to bring down blood sugar levels) it is ineffective at bringing down blood sugar levels, so more insulin is needed. When this is done too frequently over time, the risk of being overweight will be the least of a person's worries.

The pancreas that produces insulin will be overworked causing type II diabetes, which is when the insulin production is outstripped by a person's sugar intake. Our diets are increasingly loaded with carbohydrates and sugars and we eat double the amount of carbohydrates as our hunter-gatherer ancestors.

Refined sugar affects our body in a different way to natural sugars such as those found in fruit. Fruit in the bloodstream can be managed with a minimal insulin response. However, when refined sugar enters the bloodstream a significantly larger insulin response is needed to control the blood sugar level, which can increase the chance of insulin resistance.

Food has an intention

As discussed in Chapter 1, everything in existence is vibrating faster than we can ever see, feel or imagine. In other words, we are constantly in motion and our positive or negative intentions affect these movements. Through Masaru Emoto's work with water, he also proceeded to work on food sources and found that different foods also had a specific vibration.

He discovered that certain foods could be more suited to immunity, anti-stress and anti-depression, as their vibrations counteracted the negative vibrations. In most cases vegetables, fish, fruit and nuts scored the highest at helping to counteract disease, stress and depression. Chicken and duck scored better overall than other meats such as beef, pork and mutton.

He also found that cooking food in the microwave changed the structure of those that scored highly so that they became less effective. The electromagnetic waves of a microwave oven deteriorated the quality of the food and the more the food was overcooked in the microwave, the worse this became. When heating food it would seem that using the stove is better to retain the nutrients in your food than using a microwave. If you must use microwaves which sometimes I do, then I suggest limiting the cooking time to help retain the quality of the food.

In his book The True Power of Water he recounts an experiment he did with a university, when they tested the vibrations of four cooked hamburgers. The first was a microwave boil in the bag burger, the second was a homemade burger, and the third a homemade burger made with the intention of love and gratitude and the fourth was a homemade burger made with an angry intention. Not surprisingly the boil in the bag microwave hamburger came behind the second and third homemade burgers but came above the fourth hamburger that was made with an angry intention. Cooked in a microwave and a poor quality food source the first burger boiled in the bag, came before the fourth burger made with negative intentions.

In second place was the homemade burger and first was the homemade burger made with love and gratitude. This shows that foods can be made more nutritious by the words and intentions we use when we are preparing them. Just like us, they react to the world around them. Parents that cook have intuitively known this for years. After reading his book I couldn't help thinking about my Mum and the effort she puts into the food we eat when my family gather together and I considered the love and gratitude that goes into these meals.

If this happens when we are preparing food, then it is not hard to imagine that the same principle applies to when we eat. I do not have any evidence to support my own opinion but it makes sense to me, that when preparing food it is affected by our intentions, then our intentions must also affect what we are eating. If we are angry or happy those vibrations will have a chain reaction. It just seems like a reciprocal rule that if food is made with love and gratitude we should honour the maker by eating in the spirit the food was made.

Natural remedies/Super foods

Natural remedies and super food groups have their place but are not generally recognized by the medical profession as treatments per se. Although they are not chemical compounds specifically designed for a fast-acting response, they do have other qualities, they are natural, which means our bodies can absorb them easier and although they work more subtly they could be more effective long term. The point I am making is that healing takes time and your body may respond better to healing with natural products instead of strong chemical compounds.

Imagine that these natural remedies are like manure and can soak straight into the soil and crop as a natural fertilizer. On the other hand, synthetic medications are more like chemical fertilizers that are sprayed on the crops to make them grow faster and bigger. Although manure may produce smaller crops they retain the crop's nutrients. With a chemical fertilizer, the crops may be bigger but will have fewer nutrients and they are more toxic in comparison.

The same happens with natural remedies as they can be absorbed by the cell whereas synthetic medication has to be digested. The medication is targeted and will relieve symptoms quickly but we risk our internal environment becoming more toxic as a result, which can cause other issues to arise. Natural remedies can take longer to work but allow the body to get better at the pace nature intended and generally are less toxic.

List of natural remedies/super foods

Flax: high in antioxidants and anti-inflammatories/good source of omega 3

Oat: good for lowering cholesterol/source of Zinc and selenium

Bee pollen: packed with enzymes, vitamins and minerals

Ginger: aids digestion, natural detoxifier/ anti inflammatory

Kombucha: contains vitamin B and healthy live bacteria/pro-biotic to aid digestion and immune functions

Pumpkin: full of anti-oxidants and fibre/ good source of serotonin

Turmeric: antioxidant/anti-inflammatory/aids digestion

Watermelon: antioxidant good for circulation and healthy bones

Cruciferous vegetables (kale, broccoli, cauliflower, brussel sprouts cabbage): antioxidants and natural detoxifier

Hemp: protein source/contains essential fatty acids/good for muscle recovery

Lemon: natural antibacterial/high in vitamin C/balances PH level and aids digestion

Quinoa: rich in protein and fibre/gluten free

Yogurt: live bacteria, combines with the digestive tracts natural bacteria. Good for stomach and aids digestion

Dates: good source of fibre/contains minerals magnesium and potassium

Fresh mint: antioxidants/good for seasonal allergies

Vinegar: balances ph level/ good for blood sugar level control

Echinacea: good for immune responses/use for colds and infections

Nettle: packed with minerals iron and calcium. Stimulate lymphatic systems and seasonal allergies

Wheatgrass: good antioxidant and detoxifier

Hemp

Before 1950, if you went to visit a medical doctor for many aliments, they would probably have prescribed hemp oil. Back then we used hemp as medicine. In the 16th Century, farmers were bound by law to keep a portion of their land to grow hemp for the British Navy because the wood in the stem of the plant was used to make rope.

A hemp plant breathes in four times as much carbon as trees and is a fast growing plant, that produces a large amount of protein seeds. Hemp is also a realistic alternative biofuel to fossil fuels; it is a natural biodegradable alternative to plastic and can be used as an eco-friendly building material. Hemp is an incredibly useful medicine and beneficial for the environment so how is it that we live in a world where this plant has a stigma and is a taboo subject? We need to go back to the mid-20th century to find the answer.

Hemp is not to be confused with cannabis, which has a higher psychoactive THC level than hemp. This came under close scrutiny, in the mid-20th century because people were using these legal substances medicinally and recreationally. Lobby groups were formed in the USA to pressurise the government, to ban hemp and cannabis, claiming these substances were rotting people's minds. A smear campaign was created against anyone that supported the medicinal use of hemp or questioned the lobby group's motives.

Hemp was banned and production stopped overnight, for new industries to replace them, namely trees (paper manufacturing), plastics and fossil fuels. One of the real winners that stood to benefit from the ban on hemp was the pharmaceutical companies, as they were unable to patent hemp. With a ban in place, they were able to create their own patented medication as the only option.

The oceans are full of plastics, killing and maiming marine wildlife, animal species are at risk of extinction 100 times faster than in any other time in human history, according to David Attenborough. Also the Amazon rain forest shrinks by 3.8 million hectares annually, the decision to ban hemp could go down as one of the biggest capitalist mistakes against the environment in history. We are only now starting to realize the potential this plant has and its versatile uses that this plant provides for us and the environment.

My prediction is in the next few years, hemp infusions will be the future of medicine, replacing pharmaceutical medication for the likes of blood pressure, mental health issues and chronic diseases. When a therapeutic dose can be mixed with other agents the hemp could be even faster acting without causing additional side effects.

There is also substantial anecdotal evidence that people taking high doses of hemp oil in the treatment of cancer, which has caused the tumour to shrink and in some cases disappear completely. My theory on why this occurs is because the hemp helps the body switch from protection mode to growth mode, due to calming the body and the nervous system down. Therefore, immune responses are turned back on and the body can effectively remove the cancer.

Hydration

Just in the same way as our bodies need fuelling with food, we also need a daily intake of clean water to be healthy. Purified water has many vitamins and minerals that are essential to the body that is not present in the same amounts in tap water. Chemicals such as fluoride are also added to tap water with the idea that this will benefit our teeth. While I can see how brushing with fluoride toothpaste and then spitting out the paste is beneficial, I fail to see the connection of ingesting fluoride through drinking water.

When Masaru Emoto took tap water from Tokyo, he found chlorine traces which were used to sanitize it. As discussed in chapter 1 this meant that he found no crystals formed. However, when the water came from a natural source a complete crystal was usually found. Chlorine was introduced at the beginning of the 20th century in London and is just one of many chemicals used to clean polluted water so that it may become drinking water.

I believe that tap water is still safe to drink. I drink it sometimes but also drink mineral water too. I think what is more important than where your water is obtained, is that the water is treated with an intention of respect, love and gratitude. Just by doing this will help set an intention that the water is beneficial for you.

If you treat water with respect then water will respect you. Every time we drink water a part of that water will be flushed out of our body but another part will become us, within our cells, blood and organs. When we respect the water, we respect ourselves.

Ayurveda

Ayurveda means the science of life and it is an ancient Indian medicine which also encompasses Chinese medicine. It has a holistic approach which balances the mind, body and soul by incorporating science with philosophy and wisdom. When someone is assessed in Ayurvedic medicine, they are not only examined physically but are also assessed on their personality, tone of voice, mental state and digestive system. People are characterised into three body types called Vata, Pitta and Kapha.

Vata

A Vata type will typically be slim and petite or tall in build and will have cold and dry skin to the touch. When in balance they will likely be the shape of a marathon runner and would excel at endurance activities both mentally and physically. However, when out of balance they can suffer anxiety, skin problems such as excessive dryness and eczema, or breathing issues such as asthma. To remedy a Vata, natural oils are added to their diet to counteract the dryness. Vata is characterized as the element air by being light, flighty and clear.

Pitta

A Pitta type will typically have a wedge-shaped, muscular square frame and warm skin to the touch. When in balance they would have the shape of a sprinter and would excel at short bursts of powerful movements. Mentally they are focused and determined but when out of balance they can be hot-tempered and acidic. This may cause excessive inflammation in the body as the body attempts to neutralize the person's PH level to become more alkaline. This can result in boils, spots, joint swelling and autoimmune disease. The elements of Pitta are fire and water by being a fusion of heat and moisture.

Kapha

A Kapha type will typically be large-framed, prone to easily gaining weight and will be oily and cold. When they are in balance they will be grounded, caring people (often healers). If they were an athlete, they would probably be thick set and have the shape similar to that of a rugby prop (position at the front of the scrum). When they are out of balance they are prone to depression, sinus issues and are difficult to motivate. The elements for Kapha are earth and water by being heavy, dense, static and cloudy.

Once the body type and the imbalance has been identified, the Ayurvedic practitioner would then recommend suitable dietary changes which are individualized to their specific needs. For example, Vatas typically need more grounding with heavy foods, whereas Kaphas would suit lighter foods such as salads. The Pitta imbalance can be either dry or oily. Often cooling foods are recommended. It is far more in-depth than this overview, which is why it's important to have a consultation with a practitioner.

A mixture of dietary changes and herbs to aid the body's ability to detoxify and eliminate provocative foods causing the imbalance are recommended. If the body type and imbalance are correctly identified, changes will happen quickly because the body is specifically receiving what it is lacking. For every disorder in Ayurveda, there is intuition on how to resolve the imbalance based on thousands of years of experience working with diet, herbs and individual body types and personalities.

It is a holistic art form to understand each body type and how to bring their body back into balance. All diseases are not created the same way because we are all on an individual journey. Ayurveda reflects the individual needs of the person which are necessary to return them to balance.

My friend Melissa Toleman who helped me edit this book introduced me to Ayurveda, which I found fascinating from the beginning. She had first-hand experience of the power of this ancient holistic medicine. Her son came home from football one day with a swollen ankle and within the next few days his knee had swollen up too. Within a week most of his joints were painful and he was bedbound for the rest of the school term. The doctors carried out tests and started him on a course of steroids, as he was diagnosed with polyarticular juvenile idiopathic rheumatoid arthritis.

His condition worsened and so he was admitted to a children's hospital in London. The doctors suggested chemotherapy and this was the final straw for her who believed there must be another way. She carried out some research, discovered Ayurveda and very quickly they were on a flight bound for India. Her son was still so ill that he needed to take steroids with him.

In India, they stayed in an Ayurvedic hospital where they prescribed dietary changes and herbs specific to what his body required. Very quickly his condition improved and he was able to stop the steroid treatment. He went on to make a complete recovery. Six years later he still needs to be mindful of what he eats but by doing so he lives a healthy teenage life. Her belief in Ayurveda meant that she created an Ayurveda centre so that she could help others in the same way.

Juicing

One way of detoxing the body so that we can restore health or lose weight is to do a juice diet that lasts from a few days, or weeks, to a couple of months. During this period, people can survive on liquid food because natural food is churned in a blender so that they still receive everything they need without the addition of any processed foods. A typical juice diet will consist of vegetables, fruits and nuts, (preferably organic) which are full of the vitamins and minerals required to keep our cells in optimum health.

There is also evidence to suggest that juicing can help manage and often cure chronic medical conditions. If you can provide the body and cells with what they need through diet and supplementation, the body will remain in balance. Symptoms in most cases will often improve or disappear. People that follow a juicing program frequently report how much better they feel, even after just a few days.

For anyone with doubts about the power of a juice diet, there is a very interesting film on YouTube by Jason Vale called 'Super Juice Me.' In the film, several people of various shapes and sizes with serious medical problems, are invited to a retreat in Portugal for a month-long juice fast. They all start with their stories about how sick they are, how much medication they are taking and how they continue to feel worse as a result.

Once they start the programme, most of the participants feel better by day two. Jason Vale makes a good point in the film that if bananas were the cause of your health problems then you would probably just stop eating bananas. So why do people continue to eat food that is known to cause health problems?

The answer as mentioned earlier in the chapter, is that when a food contains preservatives, additives or artificial sweeteners, they change the taste and our taste buds are tricked into thinking we want more of this particular food, when in reality all we are craving is the unnatural ingredients. It becomes less about hunger and more about clinging and needing. People reach a point when they become addicted and the addiction creates an illusion that they cannot live without these specific foods.

The film shows the emotional journey of the participants and sheds light on the reasons why they are sick. Once the people start detoxing from their former diets, the cause of their poor dietary habits becomes clear. They describe the emotions they are feeling, that they would otherwise avoid feeling through eating these addictive, unhealthy foods.

The people were hiding their emotions with what they ate and when this was taken away from them, they had to face them. It was a difficult process which took them out of their comfort zones but the alternative was to stay at home cocooned away from their emotions, at the cost of their health. The retreat offered a safe place for the participants to go through a challenging but life-changing emotional process.

They also went through physical changes and in some cases, their symptoms became worse before they got better. Their digestive systems began flushing out toxins which had been stored in the body for many years and this meant they had to go through the process of detoxifying to eventually get better. Instead of masking the symptoms with food or medication, this safe place allowed them to become sick for their greater good with only natural intervention. This is a good example when symptoms are beneficial to us.

The generic juicing that was given to the group did not work for everyone. One participant in particular with ulcerative colitis lagged behind the group in terms of feeling better. His juice was changed to include only cabbage. By removing the other ingredients he started to improve.

The participants in the film were educated on the difference between foods that are alive and foods that are concentrated or processed. These foods usually have many ingredients added to them so that they can be mass-produced and have a longer sell-by date. The people were able to live this life for a month giving their bodies all the nutrients they needed. They also learnt what it felt like so that they were motivated to continue when they left the retreat. The results of all the participants were impressive, to say the least.

One participant, in particular, was morbidly obese with several underlying conditions which meant that he was taking 50 plus tablets a day. He travelled to the retreat with two suitcases, one for his clothes and one for his prescribed medication. While he was sleeping he needed a respirator to keep him alive. His posture was hunched through his mid-back with rounded shoulders, he was breathless when he talked and his face had a pale complexion. He was the poster of ill health.

After two weeks at the retreat he had lost so much weight that his clothes became baggy, he looked healthier and was far less breathless. His energy as a person had completely changed and he looked lighter not just physically but mentally and emotionally. He developed a far more positive tone and outlook. By the end of the 28 days, he was seen running up a hill which would have seemed impossible at the start of his journey.

At the end of the film, there is a review of the participants after they left the retreat many months later and it is clear to see that the retreat profoundly changed most of their lives for the better. Many of them successfully reduced their medication, started exercising regularly and replaced their old diets devoid of nutrients with healthy and nutritious foods.

Juicing is a very powerful tool when people have ill health but it is not a long term solution and is most effective when used periodically. Food needs to be introduced back into the diet at some point and if a person picks up their provocative dietary habits again, the same problems could return. It is more important to learn about food groups and understand which food groups are inflammatory to your body.

Juicing can also be integrated into your everyday diet by swapping a meal at breakfast or lunch. It is a great way to continue the good habit of eating fresh fruit and vegetables daily and for those who do not like the taste of vegetables, adding them to a blender along with a natural sweetener such as honey, makes the taste so much more palatable. This is perfect for a child who complains about not liking their vegetables. Just give them a natural daily blend of nutrients and they won't even know what they are eating!

Hopefully, this chapter has shown that the power of what we eat has an enormous effect on our health. The government is only now waking up to the fact that most chronic conditions can not only be reversed but also prevented through dietary change.

My advice is to seek out a holistic practitioner to help you understand your requirements. If you want to start making changes now then use the questionnaire from the previous chapter by changing the words "becoming more active" for "improving your diet."

Chapter 6 – Meditation is medication

Meditation can take many forms and also it could be considered that we're meditating most of the time. We just label what we call meditation by different names. The meaning of meditation comes from the word contemplation which means to think about something thoughtfully for a long time. This is why walking in nature or reading a book is a meditation for me. Often when people think about meditation they visualise monks sitting cross-legged for hours on end and believe that it is something that is not attainable to them.

Being Present

Meditation can be negative or positive depending on the focus of our thoughts and emotions. For example, going for a walk in nature, listening to music or driving a car are all types of meditation. What you think and feel during these activities will determine your experience. What if you're angry or stressed, reliving a memory of a situation or person that upset you? Or what if you're fully present observing your internal environment and surroundings without judgment? They are both contemplation with totally different outcomes.

Have you ever been for a walk or a drive and been distracted by thoughts of what someone said or reminded of an urgent task that is worrying you, and suddenly you realise you have already arrived at your destination? Being lost in our thoughts is common and is normal to reflect on our situational circumstances and our decisions. If we get stuck in our thoughts and are unable break our attention away from them, more often than not we will lack the judgement of presence of mind. We will begin to react to situations instead of making grounded decisions in reality. As discussed in chapter 1, if being present is growth mode, then being stuck in your thoughts is protection mode.

The solution to breaking the habit of your negative thoughts is simple, find a space where you can relax and take several deep breaths in and out. Allow your focus to switch from identifying and clinging, to your internal thoughts, to being the observer of those thoughts and notice how they make you feel without judgement or meaning. Over time your awareness of your surroundings will heighten, the sounds of the environment or the sensations you feel will come into focus, causing calmness. I have practised many types of meditation and this type is just as powerful as sitting still, crossed legged for a length of time.

Meditation occurs when we are engrossed in an activity that focuses our attention on reality. When we are fully present, we are only observing and making judgments based on the external environment and our intuition (feelings). The past and future has no meaning. When we focus on the natural stimuli, received through our senses, we will become relaxed. This is practising beneficial meditation.

When we strip the layers back, the goal of meditation is to help us control our emotions so that we can feel more empowered in our lives. Daily meditation can help us come from a place of love rather than a place of fear. When we are acting from the former, we are more likely to be grounded. If we are in the latter, we are more likely to make poor decisions such as seeking activities to escape the fear of our unresolved emotions.

There have been many reports of spontaneous remission in illnesses such as terminal cancer that modern medicine has been unable to explain. Through Dr Joe Dispenza's work, he discovered a similar pattern that these patients had in common. Firstly, they accepted that their mindset and how they were living their lives was the cause of their illness. Secondly, they believed in a higher power which was bigger than them. Thirdly, they practised meditation which allowed them to make changes in their lifestyle and perspective which had originally caused the illness.

We are only just beginning to scratch the surface of what is possible with meditation.

Religion

In the 21st Century, traditional religion is on the decline. Some forms of religion have been widely adopted by civilization since the day dot. Whether that was worshipping a God, the sun or the planets, people have always looked out into the world around them for guidance and inspiration. Religion has served as a self-regulating moral code for humans to live by, connecting them with others and to believe in something bigger than themselves.

Each religion has its own set of beliefs and stories of origin, but most religions unite on similar views of morality and supporting the greater good. They also incorporate practices that could be considered spiritual ceremonies such as pilgrimage, fasting and prayer. The decline of religion means that these traditions are also decreasing. However, as religious practices decline spiritual practices are on the rise.

With the rise of science and the rational enlightenment starting as early as the 18th Century, Christianity was accused of being fraudulent because the new ideas on evolution and how we came to be were at odds with a God in heaven and the miracles of the Bible. The new intellectuals were opposed to these stories and preferred to believe in a world without God.

Ceremonial worship has brought people together to sing, share advice and tell uplifting stories to one another since the beginning of tribal life. These practices provided support networks throughout the ages and are still taking place regularly today, such as people going to church every Sunday. Before the rational enlightenment, these religious rituals were ubiquitous and unchallenged in civilization.

Atheists of old had been missing out on these practices because they do not believe in a God. This means they were less likely to take part in ceremonial traditions as they believed they were of no benefits. Richard Dawkins, probably the most famous atheist rejected spiritual practices, but scientific evidence backs spiritual practices as beneficial to us, therefore, modern atheists are beginning to utilise them.

Today people have many reasons for choosing to give up their ancestral religion. When someone gives up a religious practice it can leave a hole unless it is replaced with another practice. Through studying these practices and religious rituals, science is proving that people who consider themselves religious/spiritual are happier, healthier and live longer. On the contrary people who consider themselves not religious or spiritual are more prone to feeling depressed, are less healthy than those who believe in a higher power.

As I got older I grew apart from my ancestral religion, but I've always maintained loose Christian principles as a way of life. I've always felt connected to a higher power, which felt bigger or more unifying than Christianity is on its own. My free thinking ability felt limited by organised religion because of its arbitrary nature and inability to move with evolutionary paradigms, philosophies, science and although moral, I found it was disconnected from the natural world. Even though I do not attach myself to a particular religion, I still think religion has huge potential, in the betterment of the existence of all beings and the universe.

Religion is an important part of our history and has many positive benefits. I want to make it clear that I am respectful of all religion and other people's beliefs and values. I myself grew up in a Roman Catholic family. I can attest to the unity and connectedness that religion can yield. However, I would like to see different religions become more accepting of one another instead of seeking righteousness or power. Religion is open to interpretation but the moral parts they share tend to agree on more than they disagree.

One day instead of many different churches and Gods of worship, religions could unite to develop a non-sectarian, universal church, inclusive of other religions and non-religions, while maintaining and respecting each other's God of worship. I believe this would result in less division amongst fanatical factions of religion throughout the world. If this was to happen, more people could benefit from religious practices including atheists.

This unifying principled approach would also make people of our community that we consider holy men/woman more credible. They could be an alternative solution to our inauthentic political system. They are generally empathic, community leaders that people trust. They would be ideal candidates to be included in governing decisions

 in the interest of the greater good and not only what is in the best interests of themselves.

In my opinion, the faith of any kind with a tolerance of others beliefs, is better than no faith. I prefer to believe there is a higher power or a unifying God (an indescribable vision of what that is) that connects all things and beings regardless of sectarian groups. I believe there is no division. When we strip back all the abstract concepts of society, such as the rule of laws and the monetary system, it seems clear to me, that all beings are equal.

Gratitude

Most religions have rituals of gratitude for sacred times of the year such as "Thanksgiving" which is celebrated to remember the arrival of pilgrims (English settlers in North America) arriving in America. Praying is another ritual. People pray for many reasons, to keep them safe from harm, keep their loved ones safe and to express gratitude. Praying helps to manifest what you want to happen in the same way that a businessman would set a target or goal. Families of old would have a ritual to give thanks through pray at mealtimes. When kids lose their baby teeth they pray to the tooth fairy. Showing gratitude and praying has always been a big part of our ancestor's lives.

Worshipping is another form of gratitude. Christians celebrate the birth of baby Jesus at Christmas and at Easter a remembrance of Jesus dying on the cross. If you go on Sunday to a Christian church, the priest will normally say," Let us give thanks and pray." This offering of praise and worship to a higher power is an acceptance we are part of something much bigger than ourselves. When some people discover religion it is normally when they go through a trauma of some kind. Religion allows them to believe in something bigger than themselves and that shift in focus can allow them to heal, which normally results in them feeling grateful to the God of the religion and the people that helped them. Over time they develop like-minded friends and feel part of a group. In most cases they will want to help others in similar situations. Feeling gratitude helps us see outside of ourselves and compels us to help others.

You may have heard people say that it is impossible to be grateful and angry at the same time. Like a mathematical equation, one cannot be present with the other. If you are feeling emotions then the solution is to counteract them with their opposites. It has been proven that people who focus on gratitude are not only happier but are also more popular. Science and religion agree gratitude is important and that when we are grateful we cannot experience negative emotions. I suggest writing or making a mental list of everything you are grateful for each day and observe what happens. When we focus on what we are grateful for it is impossible to focus on what is lacking.

Pilgrimage

The ancient spiritual experience of pilgrimage dates back to before conventional religion. Druidism was the main belief system in England before Christianity arrived and was based on worshipping the natural world. Instead of a God in our image, Druids worshipped the sun, the trees and anything that supported our environment. They were the original members of the Extinction Rebellion.

Stonehenge was a significant location as the altar is built to be aligned with the astronomical events of sunrise on the summer equinox and sunset of the winter solstice. This understanding of ancient astrology is noted in other civilisations, for example the Egyptians also built the pyramids in alignment (with an accuracy of within millimetres) of star geometry. It is a mystery how these monuments were built so precisely or how large rocks were moved with only the primitive technology available.

My thoughts are they were not limited to thinking in terms of how we view science today. Science back then would have been a blend of philosophy, maths and mysticism. To build huge monuments aligned with star constellations with precise calculations, they would have needed to understand that the Earth rotates around the sun. This is contrary to the beliefs of Christianity in the middle Ages, as Galileo (1564-1642) would find out. He presented his discovery to 'The flat Earther's'of the day, and they famously threatened him with execution, for which he subsequently retracted his findings.

In the modern world, we tend to look inwards. Older civilisations were not bound by limitations of modern science and modern religions, people would have been able to look up at the stars at night and know exactly the time of year it was or to observe the sun and know the time of day. Now those skills are mostly redundant because we have the use of watches and calendars, but also very few still study star constellations.

Druids used to travel as far as Scotland every year to visit Stonehenge on pilgrimage. The routes were so popular that there was a network of taverns and stop off points along the journey. Their journeys would be carefully timed to coincide with the Equinox and solstice. The significance of the site would have been a central place of worship in the same way as we now regard cathedrals and churches today.

The Camino to Santiago walk is another famous network of pilgrim trails, leading to the shrine of the apostle St James. The routes span across Europe, but the most famous is from southern France to the North-West coast of Spain. A popular film directed by Emilio Estevez has been adapted called 'The Way' starring his father Martin Sheen. The film is about an unlikely group that come by chance to walk the Camino together, to discover themselves. I haven't walked the Camino myself, however, one of my patient's has on multiple occasions and I plan to one day.

For many years my family and I would walk the Walsingham pilgrimage to the shrine of Our Lady in Norfolk, known as the Nazareth of England. There would be hundreds of people there and we would walk all day. I am unaware of the distance we walked but as a child, it felt like forever. I still know very little about the Christian significance of the shrine. I couldn't tell you the history as to why hundreds of people from around the country attended every year but I do remember feeling spiritual energy on the occasions we went there.

As a small child, I remember complaining to my Mum that I was tired and felt like I couldn't walk any further. I remember bonding with my sister and moaning about walking so much. I can recall my Dad putting me on his shoulders and feeling like I was on top of an elephant. I admired his strength and endurance by carrying me for such long periods.

These were challenging experiences but I look back fondly on them because when we did arrive at our destination, it was a relief but also an achievement.

What if there was no need to walk to Stonehenge or across Europe, for religious purposes to feel the benefits of a pilgrimage? What if every time you went for a walk you could hold the intention of a pilgrimage? Walking is one of the most natural and easy ways to meditate. Our ancestors understood this which is probably why pilgrimages came to be.

Meditation

When we think of meditation we tend to look at Eastern branches such as Buddhism and Hinduism. However, all religious traditions at some point have used meditation rituals of chanting, singing and contemplation. Christians for example use praying beads to recite mantras and prayers.

Meditation has been established as a highly effective stress reliever. So much so that mindfulness is available on the NHS for mental health issues and has been hugely successful. Meditation outperforms antidepressants for those suffering from depression. The more obvious benefits being that it has no harmful side effects and is more cost-effective.

Meditation has been proven to help the body switch modes from the adrenal, sympathetic dominate mode (protection mode), to the parasympathetic relaxed mode (growth mode). It also reduces brain activity with the brains' default mode network, which is the mode of worry and anxiety. Over time, neuroplasticity (the ability of the brain to change over time to build connections that help us, for example, learn how to play an instrument), can be moulded through meditation and control of the breath to help switch the modes.

There are two types of meditation in Buddhism. The first is the active expression of a chant or mantra and the second is mindfulness. Mindfulness is the observation of sensations without reaction in the body and has been developed in the Western world from Buddhism. It was first discovered by the Buddha Gotama, when he famously sat under a tree and remained there until he received enlightenment.

Meditation is not considered positive or negative in mindfulness. The quality of the meditation is obtained through observing sensation without reaction, whether that is thoughts of our internal dialogue or bodily sensations. It is viewing the world as it is and not how we would like it to be. There is a real authenticity to the practice. It is this understanding that helps us to bring the body into growth mode, by not clinging to wanting growth mode or the aversion to protection mode.

A God is not central to mindfulness and your beliefs are not relevant to the practice. This secular structure allows all religions and atheists the opportunity to practice together, regardless of their differences. Your experience of the practice is central to your observation of self.

Through this observation, we can connect to our inner selves and the world around us. The Chinese call this Chi. Chi is the ultimate energy source that surrounds us and connects all living and non-living matter. Through meditation, they believe your Chi is strengthened bringing you closer to Source. Chi is not a person or a thing to be worshipped but an energy field of intelligence linking everything together.

The more connected to Source you are, the more benefits meditation can bring to your life. Through these experiences, you may have insight that arises to be acknowledged and with this self-awareness, old behaviours can be replaced with new ways of being. This is why meditation can be a challenging process for some people. By going through this process of self-awareness clinging by the ego, will cause resistance to change, mainly through fear of change. If you do not become attached to the fear and instead let go, eventually the fear will dissipate and you will successfully overcome your ego's clinging.

Think of it like a fear bubble that becomes scarier as the bubble grows. If you react to the bubble it never leaves and you are left in a state of anxiety whenever you think or do the thing that causes the fear. However, if you just observe the bubble without reacting therefore, facing your fear, eventually the bubble will burst. Once the bubble bursts you will overcome fear in the mind, your body will relax and the chances are you will feel different about whatever the trigger was the next time you think about them.

This is the power of meditation. If you are prepared to do the work, by being brave and honest with yourself, you will be surprised by the possibilities available to you. A shift in perspective is the only thing stopping you from making positive changes to improve your life. I speak from my own experience of the benefits of a daily meditation practice.

It does not mean you will never become stressed, anxious or annoyed again. What it does mean is that you will be more aware of when you do, which means you will be able to modify your behaviour through response, intention and conscious choice. If you were aware every time you did something that did not serve you, eventually the unwanted behaviour will cease.

Meditation can balance and ground us so that we are better equipped to deal with stress and obstacles that life can throw at us from time to time. Processing thoughts, feelings and emotions through meditation, allows them to pass through us instead of triggering us, enabling our bodies to resist switching on protection mode and instead remain more balanced and grounded in growth mode.

A person's experience during mediation is personal to them and what they make of the experience can only be decided by them. If a person experiences an out of body experience then that is their truth and no one, including scientists, can tell them otherwise. Often there is a message in these experiences that helps the person understand their own experience and behaviour.

Meditation has been a part of eastern philosophy for thousands of years and is starting to gain traction in the west. The ability to silence the mind, to go deeper within, has many benefits and is much easier to understand than most people realise. In a fast-paced world it is a tool that is free, with no side effects that allow us to renew, helping people to re-energise, maintain a life balance and clarity on their life purpose.

Dance your prays

Dancing would have been one of our tribal ancestor's favourite pastimes. Sitting around a campfire and using makeshift instruments, they would have danced freely without feeling self-conscious of how they looked on social media or what other tribes would think of them.

It would have been a tool to release stress and bond with their friends and loved ones.

In our modern world, as we move further away from nature and the tribal way of life, we are less likely to dance and when we do dance, we are often restricted by the conformity of what others think of us. In a social setting, if someone were to just start dancing, it may make others feel uncomfortable and the person would risk embarrassment.

My first memories of dancing were with my sister in the backroom of our semi-detached house, listening to Michael Jackson's albums on vinyl. I remember feeling free to jump and move in any way that I wanted. This was a true expression of movement without any worry of what people thought of me. I only stopped when my sister put on her Bros album!

As I became older we did this less. I can't say why this was, but I guess it is because when you go from being a child to a young person you become more aware of societies norms and the stereotypes placed upon us. I remember first going out with friends and dancing in clubs. Without drinking alcohol I found it difficult to let go of being self-conscious. I enjoyed dancing but unless I had consumed alcohol I would be rigid and would laugh at others who could let go and loosen up.

When I qualified as a Chiropractor I went on a self-development course that took me on a journey to Fiji. It was an amazing experience, firstly because of the people and secondly because it is one of the most beautiful places on earth. The people are so open-hearted and kind natured. One evening on the course we had a 5 rhythm session which is a dance class with five waves of music; flowing, staccato, chaos, lyrical and stillness.

Each morning we attended a sharing group and the morning after the class a few people shared about how insightful dancing was for them. One man in his fifties shared that he used to dance a lot when he was younger but had not done so for years. He said the previous night had brought back the feeling of when he used to dance and he felt so much better and younger because of just one night of dancing.

It made me consider my own experiences of dancing with my sister as a child. It was so much fun and we often reminisce about it when we see each other. I realised that feeling good about ourselves or how young we feel is due to our age but also because of the things we do. If we stop doing the activities we did when we were younger then, of course, we are going to feel older. When I came back from Fiji, I decided to seek out a 5 rhythm class so that I could continue with my rediscovered love of dancing. I was worried that they would be hard to find, however to my surprise they were available in most big towns or cities.

I started to attend regularly and found them not only to be a lot of fun but also highly therapeutic. I discovered that if I had a problem that week or an issue that I didn't know how to deal with, I could usually dance with it and the answer would appear or the problem would resolve without action. I highly recommend it. The class does not allow cameras so you are free to be your true self. It is a safe space that is created so that people can dance freely as our ancestors did around the campfire.

Traditional Yoga

There are many types of yoga but they mainly focus on flexibility and breath work which form moving meditations. These mini mediations promote the rest and digest response (growth mode) and that is why people feel relaxed afterwards. It is also beneficial for improving posture and encouraging better mechanical movements to maintain the health of our joints.

Stretching has many benefits such as improving balance and coordination, which we tend to lose through poor postural alignment. When our joints have restricted movement we move differently to how nature intended. Over time we adapt to poor movement patterns which can result in less control of our balance, coordination and posture. Stretching helps correct these abnormalities back to their natural positions, so that we have greater control of over them.

Yoga routines accompanied by breath work can help to re-energise the body. By promoting rest and digest, the body switches to growth mode which has less of a toll than protection mode. This is why yoga is well known for reducing stress and helping people to feel more empowered about their life. When we are in protection mode we are more likely to lack clarity when making decisions, whereas when we are in growth mode we will be grounded when making decisions.

This is why breath work is so important to stretching. When we stretch we breathe deeply so that we can enter growth mode. The more we can promote growth mode, the deeper the stretch can be. Think of growth mode as stretching and protection mode as contracting. When we are in protection mode, our muscles become tight and our breathing is shallower, whereas the opposite happens in growth mode.

Each muscle group has an opposite muscle group in the body called antagonists. In yoga, the common perception is its focus is solely on stretching but the sage yogi's of the past understood that when one group of muscles are stretching, the opposite group of muscles (antagonists) are contracting. This is why yoga is not just about stretching but is equally about strengthening the body.

For example, to stretch the hamstrings you need to extend your leg and bend from your hips. In this position, the quadricepses are contracting. With practise a person can learn to strengthen the quadriceps and also stretch the hamstrings. This is how postural changes can be corrected or improved through yoga. Ultimately our posture is only a reflection of our mind and therefore if we are more aligned in our body; our mind will also become more calm and balanced.

People of any age can benefit from this non-competitive practice. Regardless of age or fitness level, yoga can be performed by anyone. Stretching can be simple and straight forward and practised anywhere. A regular gentle stretching routine in a class or practised at home will do wonders for your mind, body and spirit.

Kundalini Yoga

A few years ago I discovered kundalini yoga, which was a form of yoga used by Sikhs for religious purposes and brought to the West by Yogi Bhajan. I attended a gong bath and the teacher introduced the practice to me by saying you could attain the same results in one year that people received in ten years of Ashtanga yoga, I didn't know what Ashtanga yoga was, but what he said immediately caught my attention.

Kundalini yoga incorporates several aspects of ceremonial characteristics that our ancestors have used since the beginning of existence. This is what for me makes this practice more powerful than regular yoga. A standard kundalini class would include chanting, singing, stretching, kriyas, (holding stress positions) breath work, philosophy and meditation.

There were no classes in my local area but I found online classes and began there. I noticed the benefits immediately, at the time I was competing in Ju-jitsu and I instantly noticed the difference in my performance. Combining kriyas with breath work was particularly powerful for me because afterwards, I felt so clear within myself. There is something so rewarding and beneficial about pushing yourself further than you ever thought possible.

The pain and discomfort surface first, then the self-doubt and then the temptation to release the position. If you can continue past this critical mass of doubt, pain and temptation something magical happens. Suddenly the pain and doubt can disappear and the willingness to hold the position becomes stronger. It is a commitment to not giving up which can build confidence, not just during the kriya but also extending to other areas of your life.

Negativity can build up energetically over time within us and if we do not release them, it can spill out and affect our everyday life. For me, this has been a productive way to cleanse that negativity, so that I can clear myself and return to my purpose. It is also a great way to connect with other like-minded people. It has helped me to balance my spiritual life with the world we live in.

A brush with psychedelic to re-evaluate

Ever since humans have lived in tribes we have used plant-based ingredients for ceremonial purposes. In Peru they used Ayahuasca, American Indians used peyote and Pagans would have used magic mushrooms. Through these mind-altering substances, people have been able to heal on a deep level and reset their purpose.

With Ayahuasca, a chemical called DMT is released into the brain. This is a chemical which is usually secreted when a person is about to die. It does not mean someone taking Ayahuasaca is going to die but it does mean they will experience similar insights as if it was the case. It's been reported quite often after a near death experience, the insight gained by the individual, usually compels them to reassess their life and purpose. This is why in the correct environment, with a positive intention, these experiences can be so powerful. Through a near-death experience, we are forced to re-evaluate what is important to us.

Across Europe, spiritual circles which take hallucinogenic substances for vision quests are becoming more popular. People are working alongside shamans to uncover their unconscious patterning, so that it can help them clear past trauma and live more in alignment with their true self. Through using hallucinogenic substances people can gain a road map to explore who they are.

I have attended these types of events myself and I was surprised by the diverse community these circles bring together. I met people such as medical doctors, professionals and builders. At present these substances are illegal, so why would people from all walks of life still attend them? When I asked them many said they were not receiving what they needed from the current healthcare model and were searching for more.

People say that through these vision quests they gain more clarity regarding a problem or situation in their life. I met a woman who said she had always suffered from depression due to feelings of self-hate. She found the ceremony a difficult experience and for a couple of days afterwards felt very vulnerable. However, three to four days later she said she had the feeling that she didn't hate herself for the first time in a long time.

She said she had tried many other therapies but this one ceremony had made the biggest change for her. My own belief is that when we enter a vision quest, we release energy that has been stored within the body which cannot be removed just by talking. Through this, we can conduct an interview with our subconscious that is too deep for us to access or witness in normal life.

This cycle of confronting our fears, feeling uncomfortable by reliving trauma or past hurt but then observing the feeling passing is similar to the fear bubble

I explained earlier, regarding meditating. Releasing past trauma in a safe environment has a cross over with meditation and psychedelic substances.

A new way of judging these therapies is needed for an integrated healthcare system. Imagine a world in which medically trained doctors of the future held healing circles for their patients in the same way the shaman did for their tribe. Many doctors at present would scoff at the thought of this idea, but one day they could be, instead of treatments, performing healings. It would take a shift in beliefs to overcome the fear of this taboo but I believe one day it will happen.

As mentioned when someone has a close encounter with death they are forced to re-evaluate their lives. They start to assess what is important to them. This can result in people radically changing their lives. We have all heard the stories of people who've had a near death experience and they see the light ahead of them, which leaves them with a feeling of peace and bliss.

My Dad had a similar experience to this. He's has health issues, which means he takes daily tablets to manage his condition. His doctor changed his medication before he went away for a weekend. The new medication prevented him from passing urine and as a result, he nearly died. My mum phoned for an ambulance and he was rushed to hospital where they had to put him on a catheter while he was still unconscious.

While he was unconscious he dreamt he was floating past our local church where our family grew up and he had the feeling that my mum was inside and he wanted to be with her in heaven. This experience transformed a man in his seventies and a lifelong non-believer. When he woke he decided he believed in God and the following year he was baptised. My Dad had his reset moment just in the same way that people do, when they take psychedelic substances for ceremonial purposes.

Anyone that knows my Dad understands that he loves a story. He told everyone and anyone who would listen that he had seen the light, even though up until this point I had only ever known him to scoff at religion. How does a man cynical of all religions wake up after a near death experience and decide he believes in religion?

The answer is that when we are faced with a life or death encounter, we are forced to re-evaluate our lives. I am pleased for my Dad, as I know that people who believe in something bigger than themselves are happier, healthier and tend to live longer. For whatever reason he made the switch, science is teaching us that this decision is likely to benefit him rather than if he was an atheist that rejected spiritual practices.

More and more research shows that natural psychoactive compounds have a therapeutic benefit for us. Leading doctors within psychology are championing the legalisation of magic mushrooms as a potential treatment for depression and mental illnesses such as

PTSD. Up until recently, the subject was stigmatised by the collective authorities who proclaimed that all illegal drugs were harmful. I am relieved that professionals are beginning to realise what our ancestors have known for millennia. These natural substances could have their uses in the medical setting, when used appropriately and under supervision.

Even synthetic medications can provide insightful experiences. This has been proven with MDMA that has been trailed along with psychotherapy to help people with PTSD and emotional trauma. It has been extremely successful in helping patients to open up about their experiences more easily. There is still a stigma surrounding substances like MDMA because there is a general black and white mentality, all illegal substances are bad for us. I, however, hold a different view.

We live in a world where addictive drugs such as alcohol are legal. However, alcohol is far more dangerous to the consumer and to those around the consumer, when compared to MDMA, which is non-addictive. As I mentioned earlier in the chapter, we can successfully meditate without the use of any substances. It is the insight we receive and what we do with that insight that counts.

I am not against alcohol, throughout my life and especially when I was in the Marines, I used it to bond with friends. People often loosen up emotionally when they have had a drink and may feel safer to express feelings they bottle up. How many of us can attest to bonding with others through heartfelt conversations under the influence of alcohol that they wouldn't have had otherwise?

However, there is also a darker side to drinking, which is different from enjoying a drink once in a while to needing alcohol to escape from emotions and stresses of life. The former can very quickly turn into the latter. We can become trapped in a negative cycle because we start to believe we can only express ourselves freely after drinking.

For me, the key to alcohol is in moderation and it is there to be enjoyed socially and not as a crutch. I suggest meditating with yourself to figure out your motives for drinking. Alcohol on its own is not good or bad, it just is. I suggest if you are regularly drinking on more days than you go to the gym in a week, then it might be worth addressing your motives for drinking, in a non-judgmental way.

Although I've never attended alcoholics anonymous (AA) myself, I am aware of the 12 steps which read, as if it is the first self-help manifesto. AA isn't aligned with any sect, political orientation or organisation, but is however aligned spiritually, as one of the steps is to believe in something bigger than ourselves. When someone surrenders the limitations of their ego to a greater power they become much closer to recovering and regaining control of their lives.

There are no laws or fees in AA and everyone is treated equally. Help is only ever suggested; therefore participants are able to take responsibility and accountability for their choices. Using these principles people in hopeless situations of addiction, are profoundly transforming their lives, sometimes overnight.

What if you could profoundly change your life around overnight without needing to develop an alcohol problem first? These principles are miraculously helping the most 'hopeless' people in society, they could also help normal people. Imagine what type of miraculous change would be possible when these principles are adopted to not just us, but to our families, groups, organisations, politics and religion.

Technology

There is no doubt that technology plays an important role in our current lives today. We are blessed to live in an age where we can find answers and buy all we need at the click of a button. Information spreads so fast that we can predict and prevent catastrophes and know the scores of every sporting event instantly.

Just in the same way that a person overeats to escape reality, technology can also provide an equal distraction to avoid our emotions. Technology can consume our attention and in doing so we begin to rely on this stimuli as coping mechanism. If this happens when technology is removed we feel bored with life and the natural world. We become so engrossed living a virtual life, we forget the beauty of presence. We need to be able to use technology, but not let technology use us.

People send fewer letters and more emails today, than ever before. From a business point of view, technology has improved production tenfold. My business has benefitted from technology and I conduct most of my communication through emails and texts. However, it is important to understand what is urgent and what can wait. This way you can prioritise your tasks, allowing you to create and maintain healthy work/life balance and boundaries.

I seldom check my emails in the evenings or at weekends. I ensure that I deal with the most urgent emails during the day and if I receive replies after the working day, I wait until the next day before responding, unless under exceptional circumstances. I also leave technology outside my bedroom and sometimes leave the house without my mobile phone. I find this gives me space away from technology, so that I can use it to my advantage but leave it at the door when it is not needed. This way I make more time for nature, loved ones and self-development.

I avoid watching the news on TV because I find it is constantly searching for a reaction or fitting an agenda instead of reporting the facts. I try to avoid drama, fear-mongering and false representation of the truth. As individuals, we are safer today than ever before, we are much less likely to be victims of crime, but when you watch the news this would appear otherwise.

I take the view that if the news is important it will come into my periphery through sources I have chosen. I am only interested in reports that are written authentically and professionally. I like to read the news when I am relaxed and centred as it helps me to process better and make informed decisions and judgments. I can't do that if the intention of the news is to cause an emotional trigger in me.

I believe that films can be inspiring and good for the soul. They are like meditations, as we become engrossed in the story, which makes us feel alive. I believe a variety of ways is the key to maintaining a healthy balance. I suggest setting some time aside to watch a film that you have chosen in advance. As with everything moderation is key.

Sleep

Sleep is as important as eating. We spend a third of our lives sleeping and for good reason, as our mortal vehicles need rest and repair. When we are unwell the thing we want to do most of all is sleep. It is one of the best forms of medication. When we rest our bodies heal more quickly. Rest and repair are focused on physical maintenance during the first 3-4 hours of sleep and during the second 3-4 hours the focus is on the brain and mind.

Sleep can also be both therapy and meditation. When we dream we live out our lives through stories, images, sounds, feelings and symbols. No one knows why dreams happen. Freud and Jung both focused on the usefulness of dream meanings and symbols as a gateway into the subconscious, whereas others believe they are meaningless and are to be discarded.

I believe they are useful and when we are in tune with ourselves they can yield extraordinary insight to both self and the relationship we have with others. Not every dream can be understood but some are much clearer to interpret than others. I separate my dreams into negative or positive experiences. With positive dreams, I do not need to do anything as they mean my life is matching my dream state. However, negative dreams show me I need to start acting on something to help align the two states.

One example for me is that on occasion I have had a dream where I miss a train. This dream normally alerts me to a need to take action in some area of my life. Sometimes it is crystal clear what the change/action is and other times I have to dig a bit deeper to discover what it may be. This shows the power of dreams when you are in tune with them. They can provide valuable insight and the more patient you are with yourself, the more insight you will gain.

My pearls of wisdom

Life is a balance

In nature everything revolves around moderation. Nature has cycles of the seasons. Nature knows how to balance. When our lives are aligned with nature, they will be easier to manage and less stressful. The further away from nature the opposite will be true. Nature is connecting with others, plants, trees animals and all beings. When there is respect for nature we are exalted.

We can balance our lives through moderation and discipline instead of abstinence and avoiding. For me it's about putting life principles together that represent you and then live by them. You could lie, cheat and bully your way through life and that may get you some results, but those behaviours will also be limiting you in other areas of your life. If you live an honest life by respecting others in the short term you might not yield amazing results but long term, you will earn people's trust in a way the first example could never do. That's the power of a principled life.

It's about striving to excelling in all areas of life, instead of focusing on one or two and neglecting the rest. Let's say you're wealthy but you're overweight with underlying health conditions due to lifestyle choices. In my opinion I would not consider you wealthy. Your health is worth more money than there is in the world. If you have traded it for monetary wealth then you got a bad deal. When your goals are not balanced we focus on things that we think will make us happy or others expectation of happiness.

I suggest self-reflecting on the life you want to manifest, that will balance you and those around you, shaping the life you want and not the life you think you want. It can be a rewarding experience letting go of expectation of ourselves, to reveal a path that is usually bigger than us, which in the long term, is much more fulfilling.

Mindset

Your internal world is either your best friend or your worst enemy. You spend more time with your internal voice than any other person. Therefore you may as well get to know one another. As discussed our thoughts and feelings effect our health more than any lifestyle choices we make. Let's say someone drinks alcohol regularly and smokes but they are well adjusted vs. someone that's a 'teetotal' but they worry and punish themselves excessively. Which one would you like to be?

The first person has bad habits but they are a balanced emotionally because they are well adjusted, whereas the second isn't balanced emotionally, they don't have any 'unhealthy' vices, but their bad habit is how they treat themselves. Now in reality if a person feels empowered their vices will likely be under control, but I just wanted to make the point your emotional health is far more important than vices like excessive drinking or smoking.

Health comes first from within and is not created or manufactured by anything external to us. It's a mistake to base health on external factors. Therefore your mindset comes before anything else. We often consider that if we just change that external aspect then all our problems will go away. However in most cases we still feel the same way after the change because we never addressed the internal problem, which is more than likely the cause.

We must first realise the concept of health is not only physical but encompasses the mind and soul.

Conclusion

"The world is not dangerous because of those that do harm but because of those who look at it without doing anything."

Albert Einstein

Taking back control of your health is a choice.

I hope this book has given you a different perspective to consider when taking decisions on your health. Science and truth seeking has been diluted by the motives of the large pharmaceutical corporations. They will exert their influence to ignore certain natural truths as they cannot be patented, or inhibit them to promote medication that can be sold at significant value through pharmaceutical channels.

The domination of science and modern medicine by pharmaceutical companies has led to governments following a limited scientific belief system and created a medical system which plays into the financial interests of the pharmaceutical giants, which fund medical science. In recent months Governments (with the exception of Sweden) have been reacting to Covid 19 in ways that would seem counter intuitive, ignoring simple truths of holistic medicine that's been known for thousands of years.

Intuitively we know that keeping fit; eating well and having a positive mindset are the keys to being healthy.

My hope is that you are now in a position to make a fully informed opinion on these conventional wisdoms and decide what makes sense to you. I hope you understand that in the treatment of chronic and non-life-threatening diseases and conditions, exercise, diet and your mental health is more effective than pharmaceutical medication. You are now in a better position to understand the impact our beliefs and emotions can have on our health. Health and emotion are linked, and we have more control over them than we realise.

I decided to write this book as lockdown begun in April due to one of the UK government's biggest oversights during the initial outbreak; that your emotions and feelings affect your health. When we are fearful or experience negative emotions, we are more susceptible to a) getting sick and b) if we become sick our healing time will be longer. Our immune systems are susceptible the more fearful we are feeling. Did the Government take all reasonable and necessary measures to minimize the fear felt by the UK population?

Conversely, when we experience positive emotions like feeling optimistic, we are a) likely to be healthy and b) when we do get sick, we are likely to get better quicker because our immune systems functions at their optimum. We are gifted power over our health, which is accessed through our beliefs and emotions.

I was shocked when this wasn't even mentioned in the lockdown guidance. I was angered and saddened when the government resorted to scare tactics and punishments to enforce what I viewed as counter intuitive rules. In my view, the complete opposite of what was needed to help the nation.

I do not question the positive effect modern medicine has had on society for crisis and emergency care. I am grateful, to the people who work on the medical 'front line'. If tomorrow I was to have a serious accident then emergency care is what I would seek. I understand the usefulness of synthetic medication which saves many lives, in life threatening situations every year. However, I disagree with the dominance modern medicine has over our health practices as a whole and how far it has penetrated our overall understanding of health.

I disagree with the philosophy that the body is a machine and that we should only fix the machine once it is broken. I believe we are too often disregarding the healing nature of the body, instead using the 'machine mentality' to view the body, resorting to synthetic medication too much and too often. It is my view that synthetic medication should be used once all other options have been explored. By this I mean a holistic medicinal approach as we've explored in this book. I believe that if we were to treat the human consciousness as well as a person's symptoms, healthcare as we know it, would be transformed.

Prevention is better than the cure and prevention in many cases means lifestyle changes. It's hard to find a chronic disease in early progression that exercise or appropriate changes to diet wouldn't help. Holistic 'medicines' have been proven to slow the progression of obesity, heart disease, early onset of dementia and many other disorders.

Medicine or medication is very powerful and means more than just synthetic drugs. When we think of medicine, we might think of cough mixture or paracetamol, but what if we could all understand medicine, as the preventive action we take, like eating a balanced diet and exercising? We start to see that medicine doesn't just have to be only a pill or something we take once we're sick.

Instead of a route to lifelong synthetic medication and medical procedures, I would propose a different lifelong long medication as outlined in chapters 4, 5 and 6. I believe a more natural approach to educating patients is to teach them the significance of exercise and use motivational language specific to them. It is important that we educate people on diet and help them discover their individual body needs, and by understanding this they can eat a diet specific to them. We should help people understand that their emotions shape their lifestyles and therefore the decisions they make. In my opinion this would be far more effective in the long term than prescribing lifelong medication for chronic illness from the onset.

For years the counter argument to revolutionise the healthcare service away from the disease centric model, has always been argued that the cost of investment would be prohibited, but the UK government has borrowed more money this year than Gordon Brown borrowed in 10 years. Investing to develop a healthcare system that was proactive and 'cause' centred, would cost a fraction of what the government has spent during this pandemic.

For me, the biggest impact on humanity in the 'new normal' is the loss of our freedom of speech. Throughout this process anything other than the government's narrow view on the subject has been censored or labelled as conspiracy theories. Democratic politics is about encouraging debate and being accepting of other people's views even if we disagree with them. Removing those that oppose you by discrediting without addressing them, results in weak and polarizing politics.

Freedom of speech is what underpins the liberal democracies, we have sought and fought to uphold. It is, without question, as significant as saving lives in the long run. Our parents and grandparents gave their lives in the name of the political systems that we live under in modern times. How can we find our true purpose if our freedom to express ourselves is dictated by the few? We are in danger of living a digital dystopian future that books and films have warned us about since the Second

World War; a war that was fought to protect our freedoms.

I fear that the deception of false patriotism such as "save our NHS" causes apathy amongst so many, as well as causing political naivety. The general public, through absolute lack of choice and voice, is being forced into a regime that is ever more similar to that of China. Just one year ago, this would have seemed unfathomable. With more and more civic freedoms removed it is time to say 'enough is enough'. In the beginning they had the excuse that time was short but six months on to still be passing laws by decree such as the 'rule of 6' is in my view unacceptable in a democratic society.

To top this off the government is telling us this is our fault, the general public because we are struggling to adhere to new policies and rules we never asked for or voted in and encouraging blame culture so that people tell tales on one another. Divide and conquer.

I understand some of the views in this book go beyond what science is willing to accept at present. I feel it's important to reaffirm that science is a discovery, not an invention. When we wait for science to discover what the sages of the past already knew, intuitive truths that live inside all of us are negated.

When Buddha sat under a tree until he became enlightened he predicted the quantum field. He described tiny little particles that were in constant flux. The Greeks were the same, they also proclaimed that

that the smallest particles were not solid and were moving. How did the sages of the past know this without instruments or microscopes? In my opinion they were clearly tapping into their intuitive senses, which were not blunted by limiting modern paradigms.

Science has brought us great advances. The path to truth and knowledge brought about in rational enlightenment has accompanied an improvement in our standard of living, life expectancy and extraordinary discoveries. However modern science is a paradigm that has become exempt from critical thinking and sceptical investigation.

We are too reliant on the few in authority, such as SAGE members, dispensing their judgments from narrow belief systems, discarding other factors irreverent, other than the scientific evidence they choose. This closed mindedness by those controlling science, by virtue is making science a dogmatic process instead of an evolving philosophy.

In Rupert Sheldrake's book, Science set free, he references polls suggesting we feel disconnected and untrusting of science because of these reasons. People in the polls often said "science is driven by business" or assume "it's all about money". Everyday people are forced to place huge amounts of trust in the scientific process, however counter intuitive that may feel to them and therefore they understandably feel sceptical.

In the 1960s the science was becoming clear that heavy smoking was not good for our health. With vested interests to combat these claims the tobacco companies funded their own research to counter these claims developing a strong body of conflicting research that they used to defend their products. They were taken so seriously that anti-smoking legislation was delayed for many years. It would appear there is good science and there is bad science and currently normal people are at the mercy of this dichotomy.

Why are we not including our smartest philosophers, artist and intellectuals in the scientific debate? Science on its own is important but without these other components is also limiting. If we were to combine other modes of thinking to gel with our scientist's, I believe human progress would be greatly enhanced.

Over £1,000 billion is spent worldwide on scientific research annually. What if a small proportion of that budget was used to fund alternative holistic science? What if for every pharmaceutical study, a small proportion of funds went towards a developing holistic science? If there was no monetary gain, what would science look like? I'm guessing there would be fewer new pharmaceuticals medication on the market and in its place, innovative and holistic approaches.

Science like the universe itself is evolving and to stay relevant with human progress, supporters of science need to be more tolerant of other people's world view. Only by openness to other modalities over dogmatism can we rediscover the wisdom of ancient civilizations and reclaim our common sense.

"In many shamanic societies, if you came to a medicine person complaining of being disheartened, dispirited, or depressed, they would ask one of four questions: When did you last stop dancing? When did you stop singing? When did you stop being enchanted by stories? When did you stop finding comfort in the sweet territory of silence?"

Gabrielle Roth (5 Rhythms founder)

Our Health Is Our Responsibility

We as individuals need to play our part by educating ourselves about health, philosophy and psychology. Instead of waiting until we are already sick to approach the health service and then expecting to be fixed. Just like we would take a car to a garage when they breakdown.

This century our healthcare must extend beyond symptoms if we are to progress. Healthcare needs to acknowledge we are a product of nature with emotions and feelings that dictate the state of our health. Healthcare providers need to be grounded in science but also philosophy and the art of living.

We all know a doctor that knows us extremely well, that doctor lives inside of us. This doctor is listening, feeling and assessing everything that happens within our bodies and tells us subtly or through symptoms like pain. Our bodies are constantly talking to us. The more we can understand our own health, the more we are in control.

Why we are here is life's mystery. The fact is as conscious human beings we are gifted a life on earth, regardless of the reason. Every breath we take is blessing, although more often than not we take this life for granted. The 70 -100 trillion oceanic universes of cells that live inside of us, that come together to make us, us, their existence depends on those very breaths.

We are here only because the sun rises every day and the moon rises every night. There are so many chance variables that had to happen for life to flourish here on earth. I feel truly blessed that those chances events happened and that "I am". The sequence of events for us to be alive now, in this time, for a tiny period of existence, in the existence of the entire universe is not lost on me and I hope that you feel the same.

Final words

Contrary to my views in this book on lockdown, I personally got a lot out of the time. I wrote this book for instance. Like most people, I had time to slow down and consider my life. I feel because of the detachment from normal life I gained insight beyond my years, which I might never had obtained otherwise. Life for me is about making the best of the time with the cards we are dealt.

Take the time to learn more about yourself and your emotions. In the beginning this will be difficult because when we pay close attention to them they might scare us, but know they are only giving you information, about how you feel and like every emotion, they will pass. Over time allowing them to surface through being honest with yourself, you can identify and decide on how best to resolve them. Understanding your emotions is a skill, it takes time and courage, but if you're prepared to do the work, the results will empower you.

I hope this book has given you more confidence to become your own authority on matters relating to your own health. By taking responsibility of your health you will start to understand yourself and therefore be able to act on your own personal circumstances. To break the cycle, we need to 1) spot the warning signs 2) be proactive and 3) courageous enough to believe in our decisions in spite of potential resistance. Listen to your inner voice and feelings to make decisions that make sense to you, as well as seeking advice from a primary care practitioner that is aligned with your values.

The fact is, we are not immortal, one day, each and every one of us will die but the good news is that we've some control over how we die, by the choices we make throughout our lives. I hope this book inspires you to learn more about your own health so that you can take control of your life instead of someone else controlling it for you.

Whatever you believe happens after death no one knows and if someone says they do, then it's only their interpretation, their belief, which they are entitled too. The clock on your mortal life is ticking from the day we are born. Make use of the time.

I would like to end with this...

Your time is now and can only be now. As adults our health is our responsibility and we need to learn about health, to maintain this responsibility. Changing your health is your choice and only you can make that decision.

Go well fellow being.

Recommended Reading

Science set free by Rupert Sheldrake

The vaccine book by Robert Sears

Dissolving Illusions by Roman Bystrianyk and Suzanne Humphries MD

The Hidden Messages of Water by Masaru Emoto

7 Habits of Highly Effective People by Stephen Covey

Unthered Soul by Michael Singer

Power vs Force by David R Hawkins

How to Eat, Move and Be Healthy by Paul Chek

A Short History of Nearly Everything by Bill Bryson

Online resources

Un-doctored- Dr Willian Davis

Chek institute- Paul Chek

Kundalini live: https://www.kundalinilive.com/

Toby Young: https://lockdownsceptics.org/

Lockdown stats: http://inproportion2.talkigy.com/

Dr Sherri Tenpenny's website: https://vaxxter.com/

Graphs from chapter 2 can be found:
www.dissolvingIllusions.com

About the Author

David Tennison's life journey took him from being in the Marines, to a civilian career that begun in the fitness industry. In that time he was gifted the opportunity to work on a pilot project within the NHS as an Activity Specialist. During these experiences he learnt insights that are covered in this book.

He is an independent thinker, questioner of systems and processes so that they can work for the greater good. He has a strong passion to support others take control of their health through lifestyle and understanding holistic principles.

He is currently practicing as a Chiropractor but is not limited to Chiropractic.

Social media links:

Facebook:
https://www.facebook.com/TheBackDoctoruk
Instagram: The Back Doctor UK
Twitter: The Back Doctor UK

Printed in Great Britain
by Amazon